An Illustrated

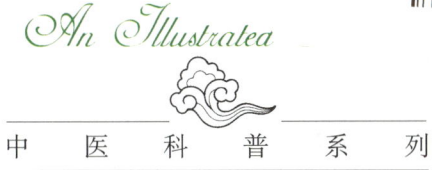

中 医 科 普 系 列

糖 尿 病

How Can Chinese Medicine Help My Diabetes?

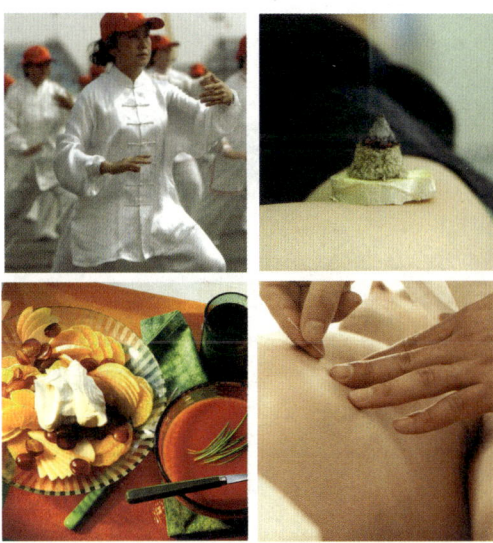

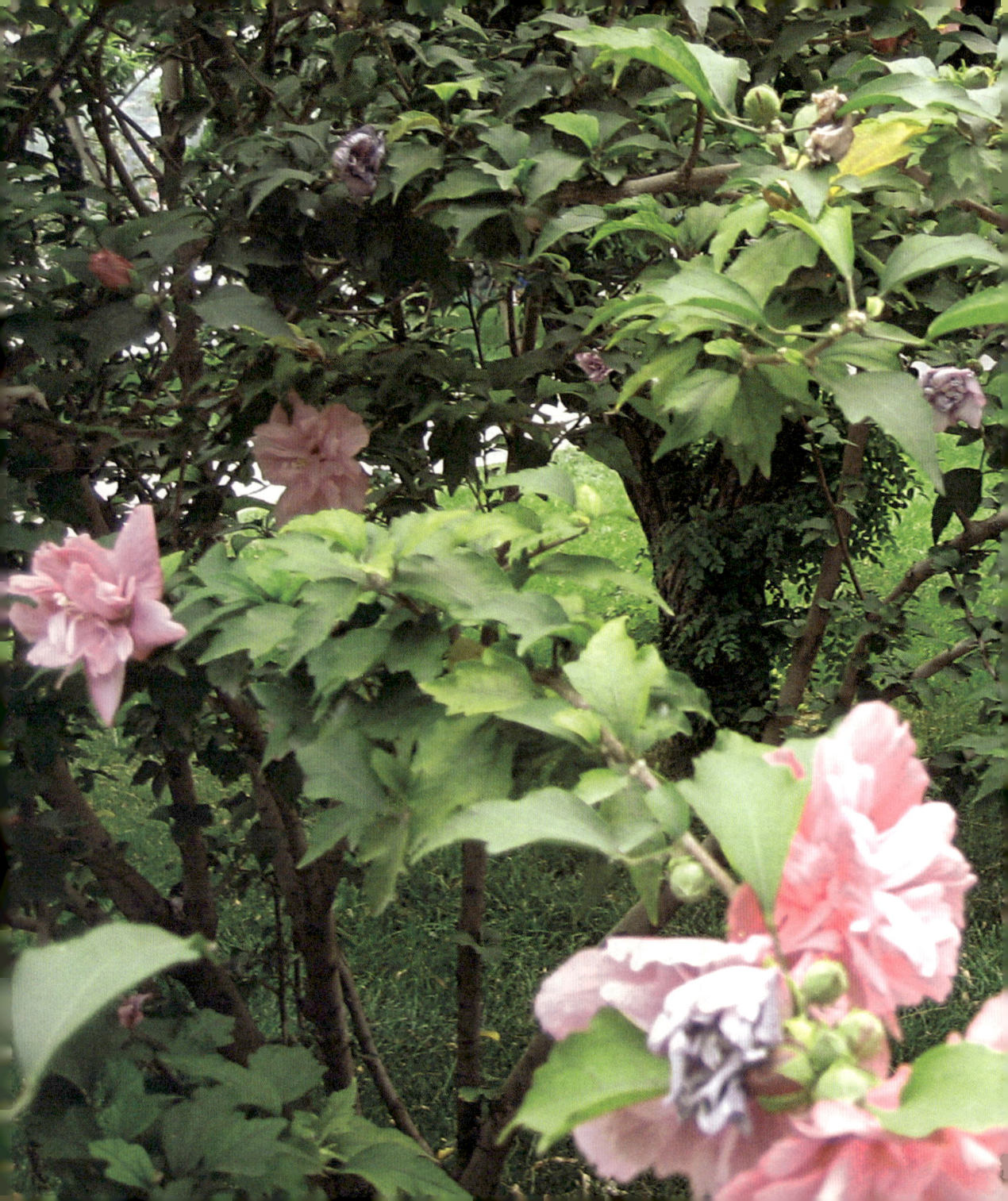

An Illustrated Guide

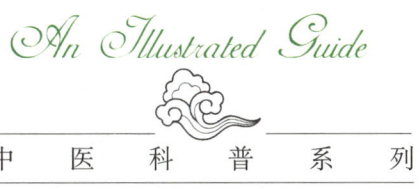

中医科普系列

糖 尿 病

How Can Chinese Medicine Help My Diabetes?

Li Xiao-li Ph.D. TCM
with Co-author: **Carl Stimson**, L.Ac.

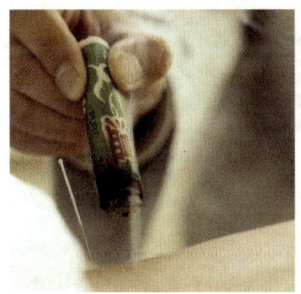
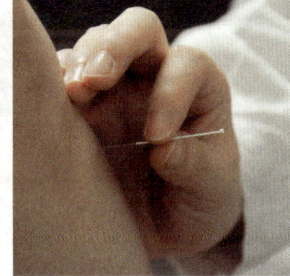

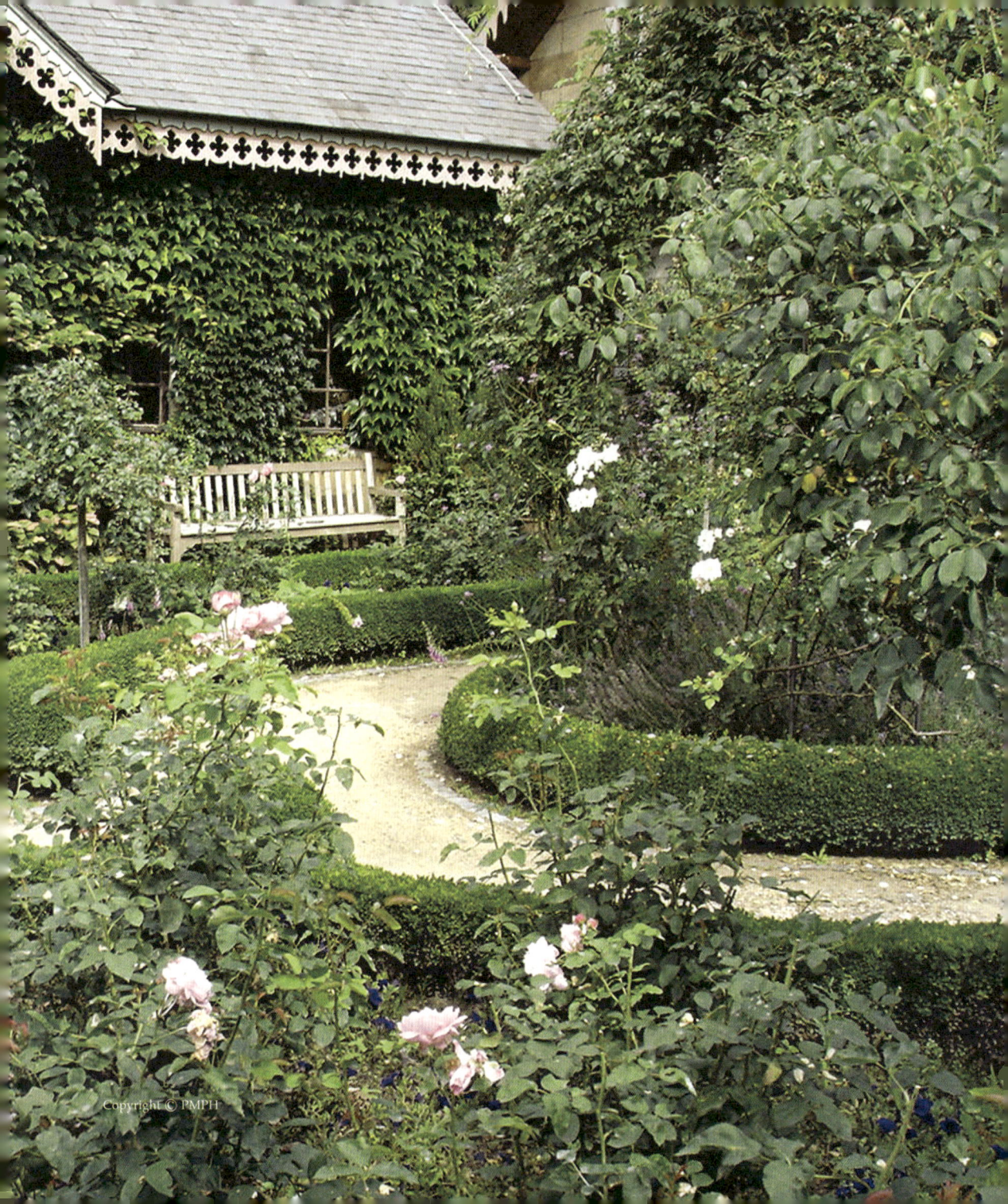

An Illustrated Guide

中 医 科 普 系 列

糖 尿 病

How Can Chinese Medicine Help My Diabetes?

Edited by Carl Stimson & Zhang Nai-ge
Illustrated & Designed by Beijing Duanzhi Shiji Advertising Co., LTD

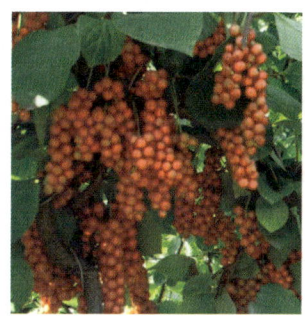
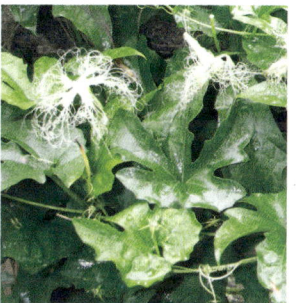

PMPH PEOPLE'S MEDICAL PUBLISHING HOUSE

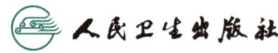
Website: http://www.pmph.com

Book Title: How Can Chinese Medicine Help My Diabetes?
— An Illustrated Guide
中医科普系列——糖尿病

Copyright © **2008** by People's Medical Publishing House. All rights reserved. No part of this publication may be reproduced, stored in a database or retrieval system, or transmitted in any form or by any electronic, mechanical, photocopy, or other recording means, without the prior written permission of the publisher.

Contact address: Bldg 3, 3 Qu, Fangqunyuan, Fangzhuang, Beijing 100078, P.R. China, phone/fax: 86 10 6761 7315, E-mail: pmph@pmph.com

Disclaimer

This book is for educational and reference purposes only. In view of the possibility of human error or changes in medical science, neither the author, editor nor the publisher nor any other party who has been involved in the preparation or publication of this work guarantees that the information contained herein is in every respect accurate or complete. The medicinal therapy and treatment techniques presented in this book are provided for the purpose of reference only. If readers wish to attempt any of the techniques or utilize any of the medicinal therapies contained in this book, the publisher assumes no responsibility for any such actions.

It is the responsibility of the readers to understand and adhere to local laws and regulations concerning the practice of these techniques and methods. The authors, editors and publishers disclaim all responsibility for any liability, loss, injury, or damage incurred as a consequence, directly or indirectly, of the use and application of any of the contents of this book.

All images in this book solely belong to Duanzhi Shiji Advertising Co., LTD, except those marked with Copyright © PMPH, the copyright belonging to People's Medical Publishing House.

It was impossible to contact the author for some images in this book, if you are the genuine owner of these images, please contact Duanzhi Shiji Advertising Co., LTD, they will pay for the use of these images.
Phone: 8610 6763 3273, E-mail: aijing129@163.net

First published: **2008**
ISBN: 978-7-117-09119-0/R·9120

Cataloguing in Publication Data:
A catalog record for this book is available from the CIP-Database China.

Printed in P.R. China

Foreword

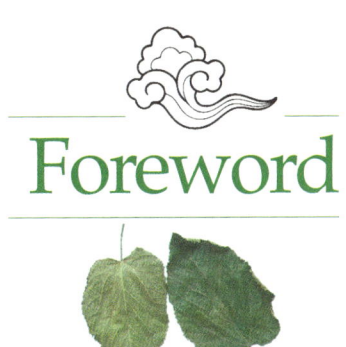

Diabetes mellitus, a common chronic metabolic disorder, has imposed tremendous suffering on the modern world. The number of cases globally has dramatically increased in recent years and will continue to rise in the future, especially among cases of type II diabetes. According to World Health Organization estimates, at least 177 million people worldwide suffer from diabetes and this figure is likely to more than double by 2030. Already, around 4 million deaths every year are attributable to the complications associated with diabetes.

Modern medicine emphasizes prevention since diabetes inevitably progresses and is extremely costly once a patient is diagnosed. After diagnosis the focus is on comprehensive disease management primarily using pharmaceutical drugs. However, biomedical treatment alone is unable to solve the fundamental problem. Sooner or later, most diabetes patients will die of complications related to their disease. These complications are actually more damaging and painful than the disease itself. Today millions are suffering from blindness, kidney failure, strokes, heart disease, amputations, and premature deaths due to diabetes.

Chinese medicine has long recognized, understood, and treated diabetes mellitus. For thousands of years its methods have been widely used and practiced, spreading in recent years to countries around the world. Chinese medicine is best characterized by its natural philosophy of healing the body, which serves to guide all of its treatments. This philosophy understands the complex workings of the natural world and uses these principles to adjust the imbalances that are the source of disease. It is far more than a traditional or folk healing practice. It aims to improve the body's overall function, slow the progress of disease, prevent complications, improve the quality of life, and prolong the life span.

This book has been written and compiled to introduce patients to the treatment of diabetes mellitus in Chinese medicine. It hopes to provide another horizon for those who are open-minded and willing to see the world differently. It seems you are one of them since you opened this book.

Guide to the Book: What Can This Book Do for Me?

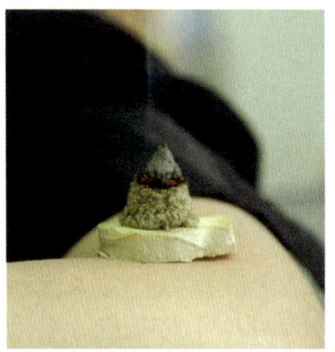 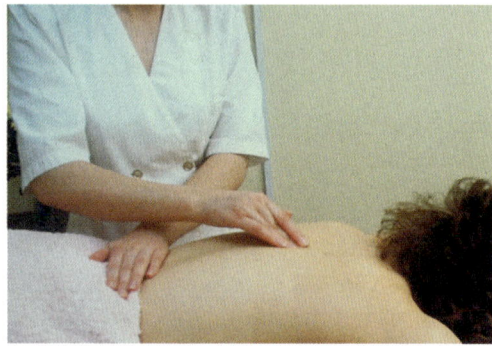

This book is designed to accomplish two things for YOU.

Explain

You may be considering treatment for diabetes mellitus with Chinese medicine but you have no idea what treatment will be like. Or you may have already begun treatment and want to know more about the theories and methods used and participate in the changes happening to you. If you find yourself in one of these situations, then this is the right book for you. It will help you to better understand what Chinese medicine is, how it can help, and what is involved in treatment. The basic theories will be introduced and the methods used by practitioners around the world will be explained in detail. Explanations of commonly known techniques such as acupuncture and herbal medicine, as well as lesser known modalities like moxibustion and tui na (massage), will help clear up any questions or misconceptions as well as prepare you for treatment. And lastly, where available, excerpts from modern research and clinical trials are included to inspire confidence in the ancient theories and methods.

Guide

The second purpose of this book is to provide you with a resource that can be used to help implement lifestyle changes that will alleviate symptoms as well as increase general health and prevent future illness. There is helpful information on eating habits, exercise programs, and a variety of at-home treatments that are both easy and affordable. From experience, doctors of Chinese medicine know that with proper treatment the amount and intensity of biomedical intervention necessary can be reduced or even eliminated. It is our hope that with the help of this book as a guide, all kinds of medical intervention can be reduced so that your time, energy, and money can be better spent doing the things you love.

While there is a lot of valuable information in the following chapters, this book is in no way intended to substitute for the care of a trained professional. Making a proper diagnosis and prescribing effective treatments are skills that take years to master and is especially difficult in complex problems such as diabetes mellitus. Chinese medicine is a highly individualized system, and the help of a proper guide, especially in the beginning stages of treatment, is essential. For suggestions on how to go about finding a qualified practitioner of Chinese medicine, please see Appendix 4.

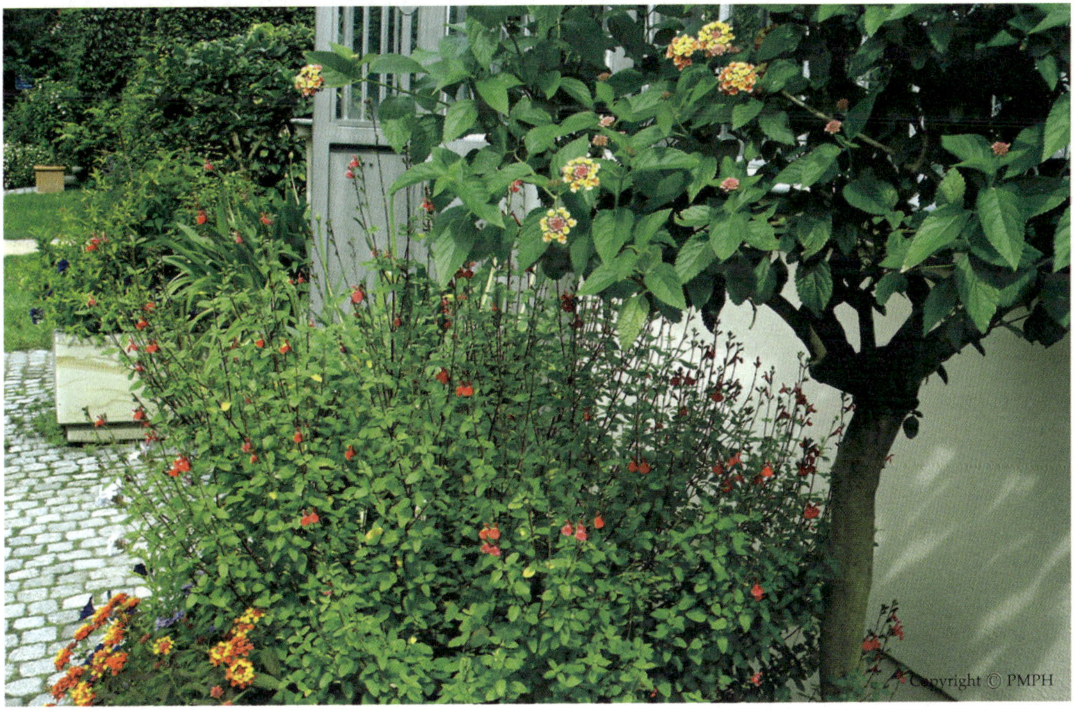

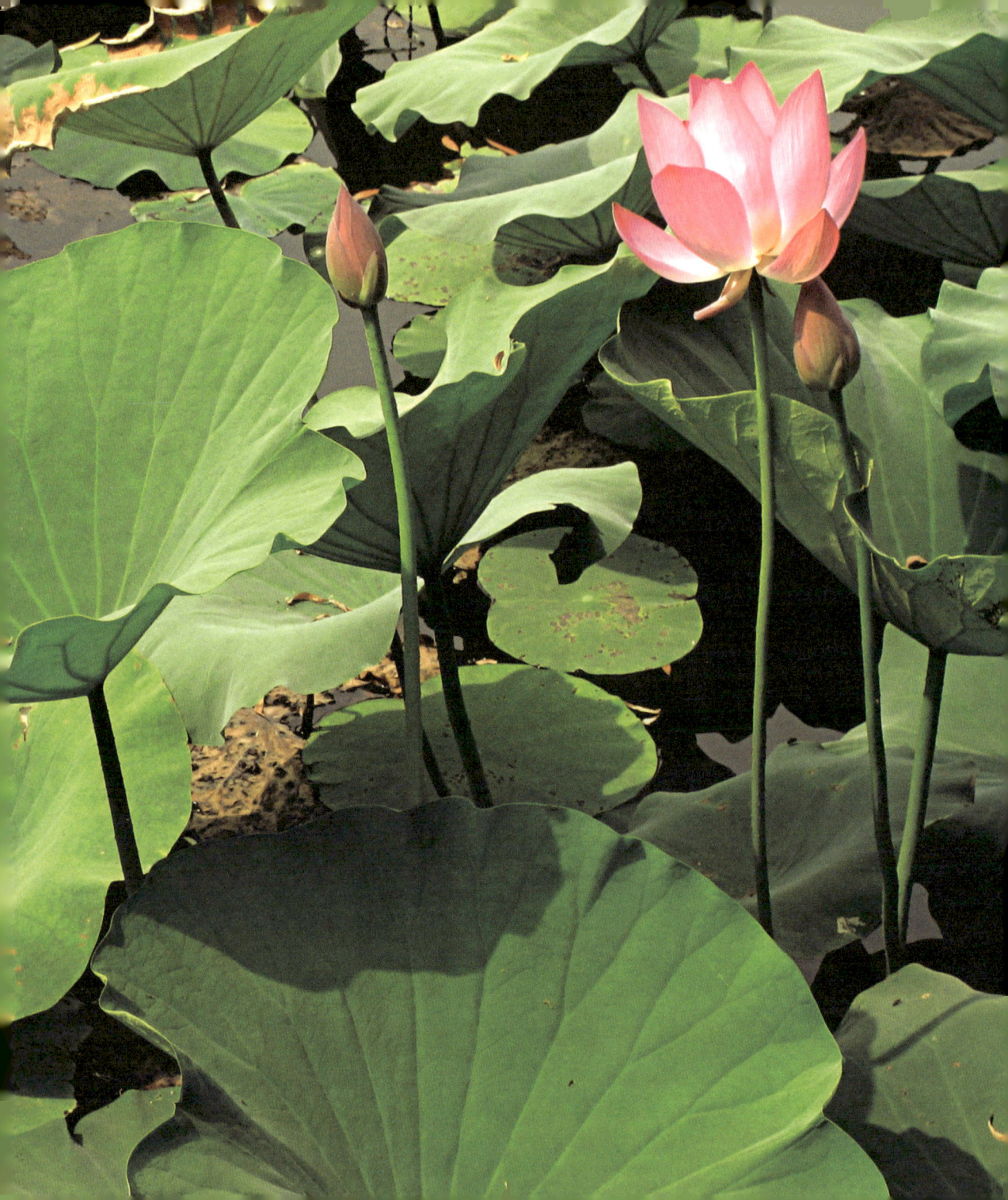

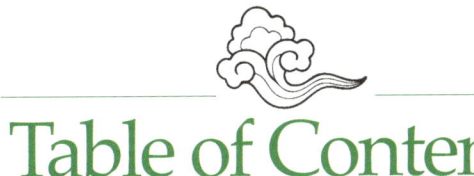

Table of Contents

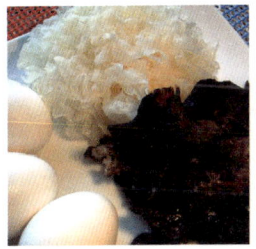 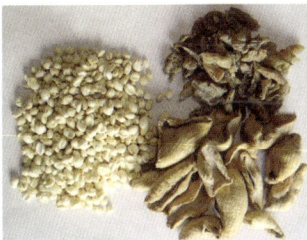 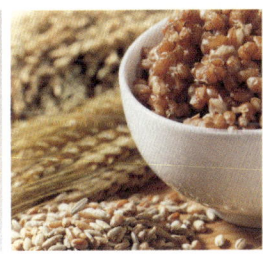 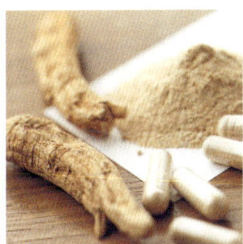

Chapter 1   Why Chinese Medicine?   3

Chapter 2   How Does Chinese Medicine Understand Diabetes Mellitus?   11
    Introduction to Chinese Medicine   12
    Two Key Concepts in Chinese Medicine   15
      1. Qi   15
      2. Yin-yang   23
    Diabetes Mellitus in Chinese Medicine   29

Chapter 3   How Can Diabetes Mellitus Be Prevented?   37
    Diet   40
      1. Essentials of Chinese Dietary Theory   41
      2. Specifics and Recipies for Diabetes   44
    Exercise (Tai Ji Quan,Qi Gong)   57
      1. What Kinds of Exercises Are Helpful and What Should Be Avoided?   57
      2. Tai Ji Quan and Qi Gong   58
      3. Translated Research   64

Chapter 4   How Does Chinese Medicine Manage Diabetes Mellitus?   67
    Acupuncture and Moxibustion   70
      1. What Is Acupuncture and Moxibustion?   70
      2. How Does Acupuncture Work?   73
      3. What Will My Treatment Program Be Like?   84
      4. Translated Research   88

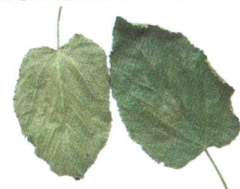

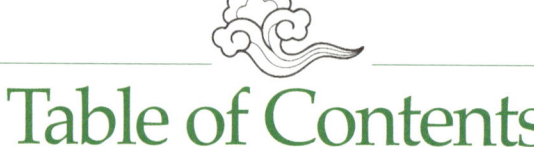

Table of Contents

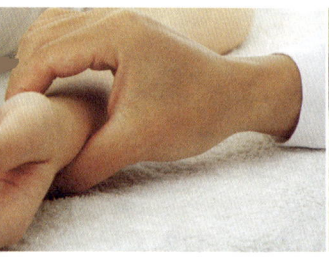 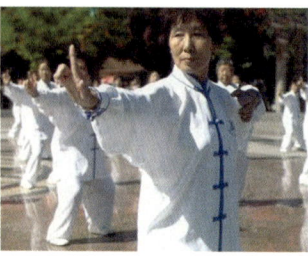 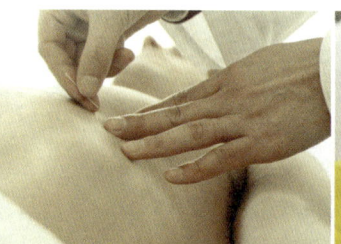 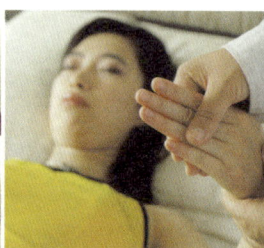

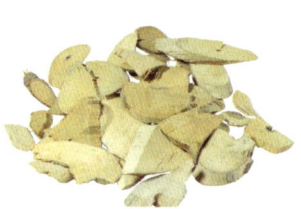

Chinese Medicinals 90
    1. What Are Chinese Medicinals? 90
    2. What Will My Treatment Program Be Like? 100
    3. Translated Research 109

Tui Na (Massage) 111
    1. What Will My Treatment Program Be Like? 112
    2. At Home Massage 114
    3. Translated Research 122

At -Home Therapies 124

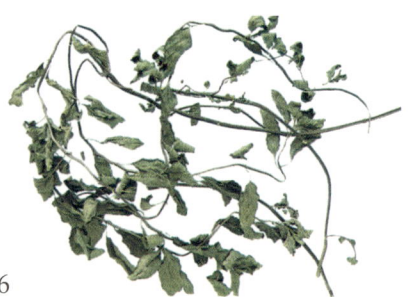

Chapter 5   Case Studies 131

Conclusion 141

Appendix 145
    1. Basic Disease Information (Biomedicine) 146
    2. Global/National Statistics 148
    3. Additional Reading Material (Disease Specific, General Chinese Medicine) 153
    4. How to Find a Practitioner of Chinese Medicine? 154

Reference 156
Index 164

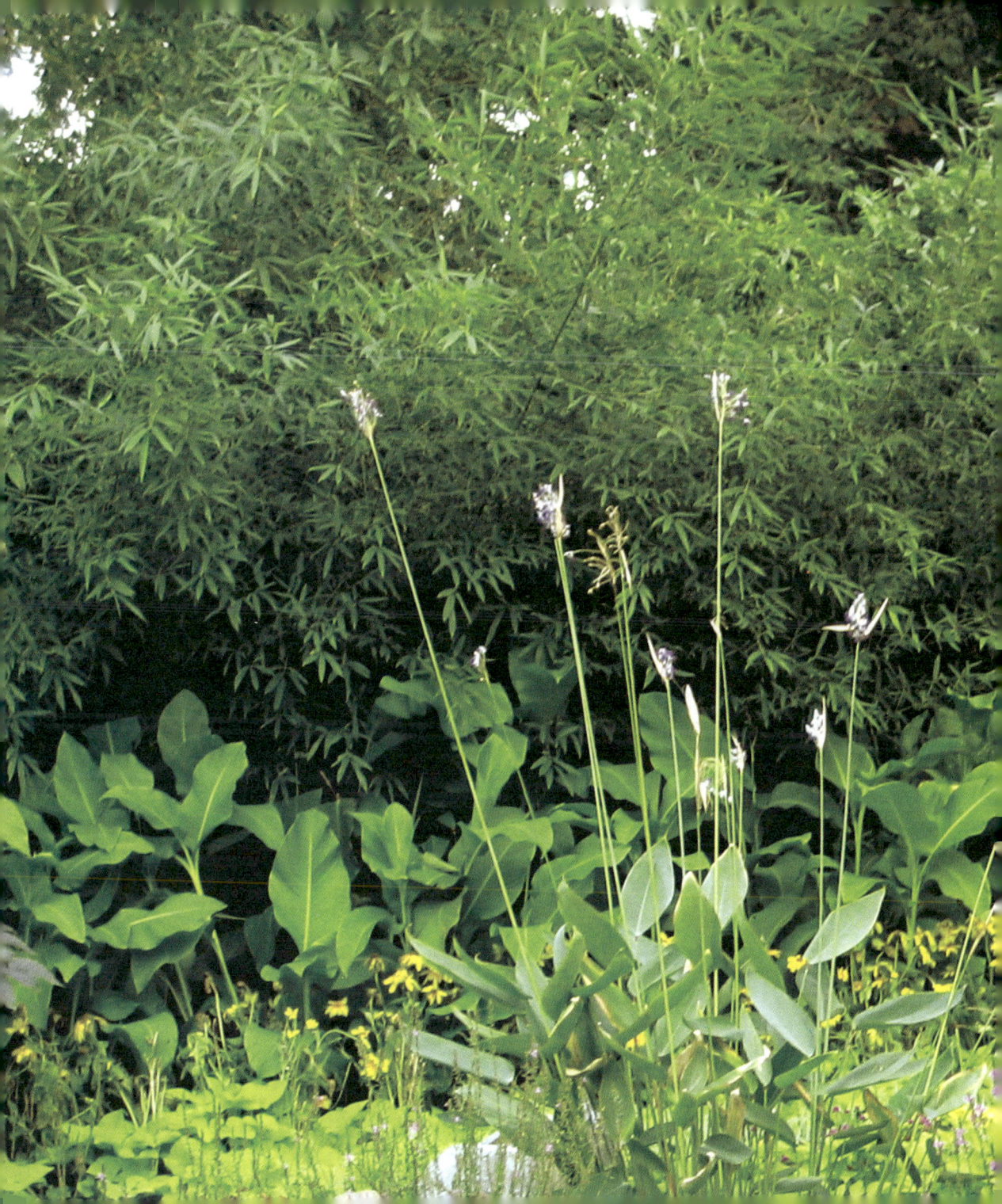

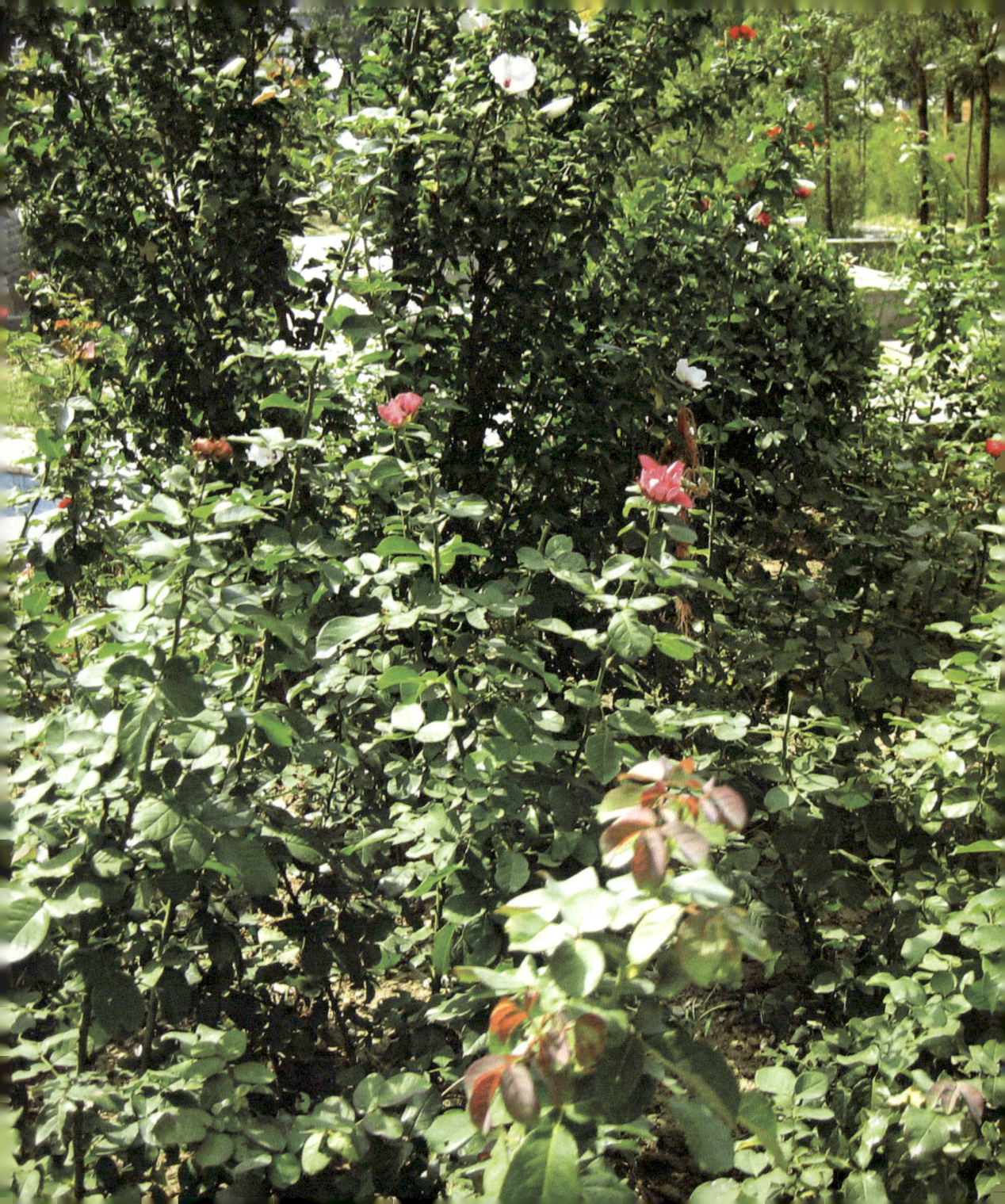

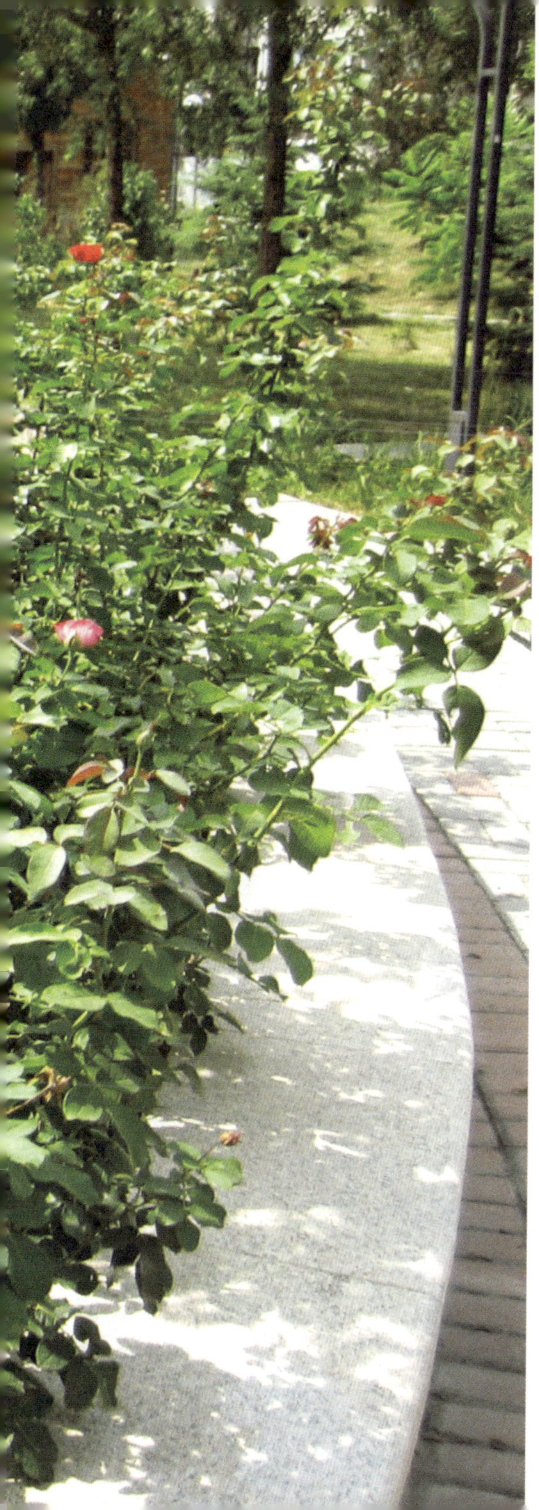

Chapter 1

Why Chinese Medicine?

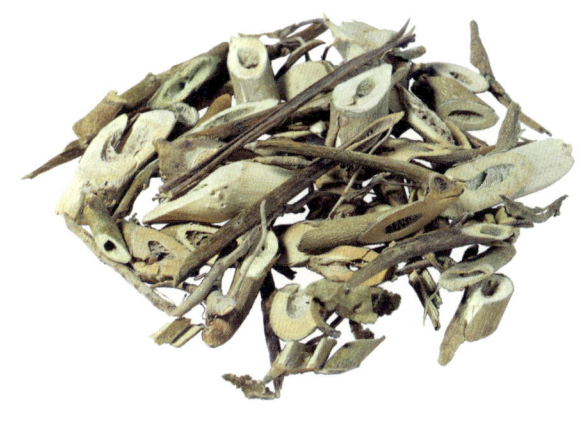

Why Chinese Medicine?

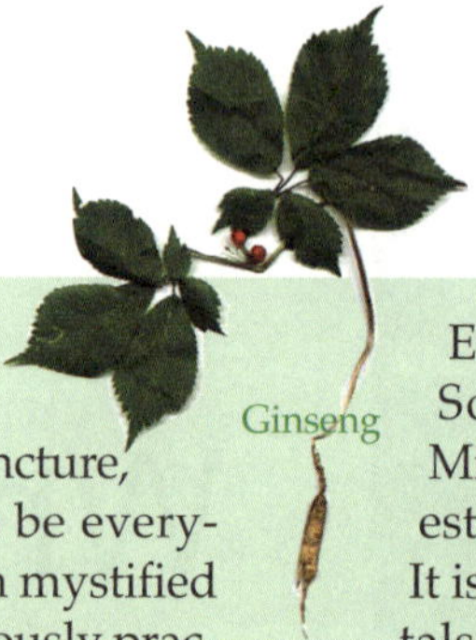

Ginseng

Without a doubt you have been hearing things about Chinese medicine for some time now. Acupuncture, tai ji, and yin-yang theory seem to be everywhere recently. An ancient and often mystified art, Chinese medicine has been rigorously practiced for thousands of years. In recent times it has been well received by people in different countries all over the world. There are well established schools all over North America and Europe as well as a growing field in South America, Africa, and the Middle East, not to mention its firm establishment in all Asian countries. It is not unusual these days for hospitals in major cities to employ practitioners of Chinese medicine and many insurance companies are choosing to cover treatments due to its efficacy, low cost, and safety.

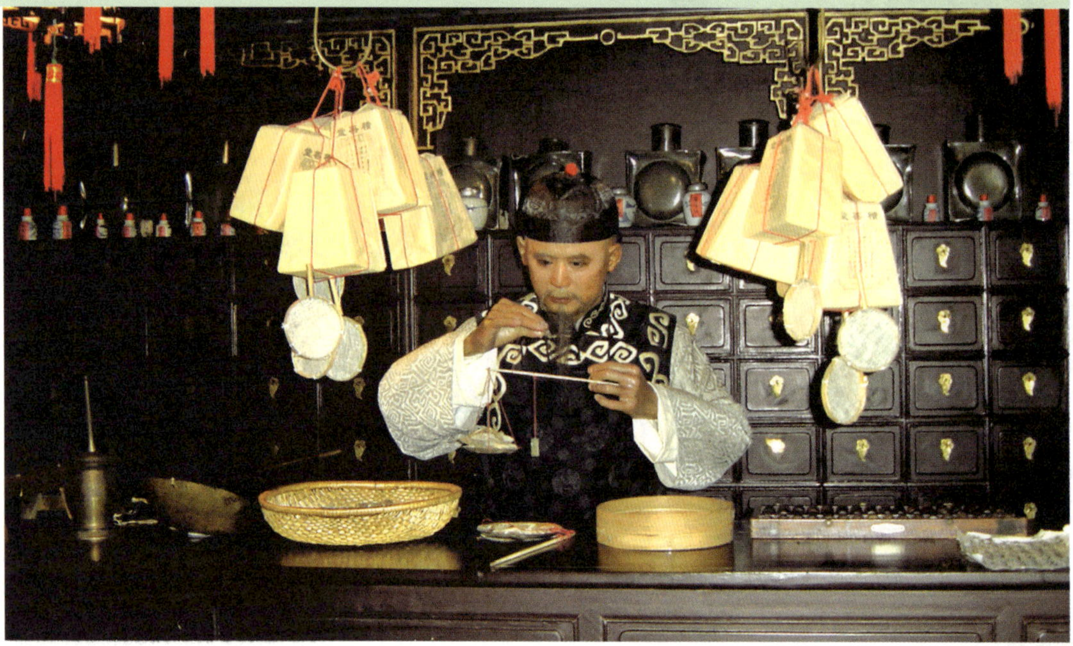

For most people who have grown up with biomedical treatment, it is difficult to resist comparing Chinese medicine to biomedicine. Most people outside of Asia still do not consider it a true scientific medical practice according to modern standards and criteria.

Despite the temptation and tendency to do so, Chinese medicine should not be compared across the board with modern biomedicine. To quote Judith Farquhar from her lecture in Beijing, 2005, the comparision "should engage with realities more than with ideals". Before comparisons are made, one should be familiar with each system. Though evaluation of the efficacy of Chinese medicine needs to be up to par with modern research standards, there are fundamental differences between Chinese medicine and biomedicine that lie outside the realm of lab tests and clinical trials. The two systems are different in terms of their philosophy, principles, and approach to treatment. As you read this book, we hope you can begin to understand the power and subtly the Chinese system has to offer.

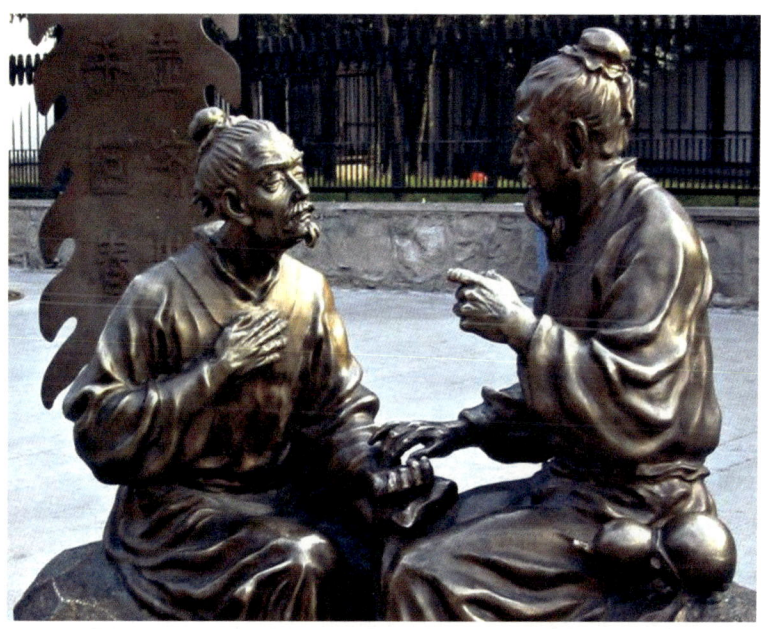

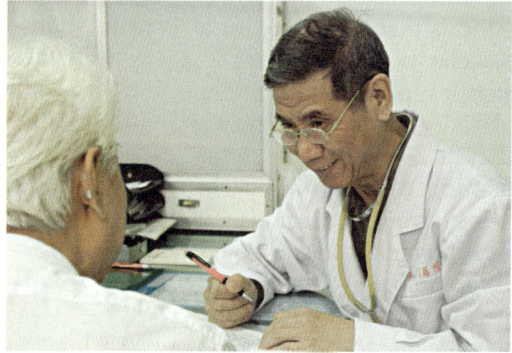

Zhou Ping-an, Professor of Beijing University of Chinese Medicine

Chinese medicine can offer a transformational experience for those who suffer from diabetes or any other disease. It is more than decreasing your blood sugar level. It is about recovering your natural ability to heal; relieving discomforts which may not go away even if your sugar levels are normal; improving your quality of life, maximizing your sense of well-being, eliminating or delaying complications, and achieving a longer and happier life.

While biomedical treatment thrives in emergency rooms and during surgery, it seems to lose its power when faced with the many chronic diseases plaguing modern society, especially diseases like heart disease, stroke, cancer, diabetes, and lung disorders that are now labeled the world's leading killers by the WHO. With diabetes specifically, the problem lies primarily in a lack of a comprehensive treatment plan and lifestyle management program. One has to wonder if biomedicine is really capable of comprehensive treatment, or merely claims to?

Administering pharmaceuticals that substitute for a weakened bodily function or artificially replace an insufficient substance can make a patient's laboratory results look better and may even make the patient feel better, but often come with uncomfortable side-effects and lead to difficult complications over time. Many drugs for diabetes are intended to be taken for life. Therapies such as these are clearly not aimed at restoring the body's own ability to maintain health.

To list some examples, sulfonylureas (like orinase, tolinase, glucotrol) can stimulate insulin release from pancreatic β cells, yet they work on the assumption that the prancreatic β cells are functioning well. In reality, diabetic patients either have a non-functioning pancreas (type I) or pancreatic cells that gradually become less effective (type II). Using this drug will temporarily reduce blood sugar levels, but it burdens the remaining "normal" cells, accelerating the collapse of the pancreas. Biguanides (like glucophage) alter insulin action by increasing the body's uptake of sugar, thus decreasing blood sugar levels. It tends to lower both fasting and after-meal sugar and trigleceride levels in obese diabetics without the weight gain associated with insulin or sulfonylurea

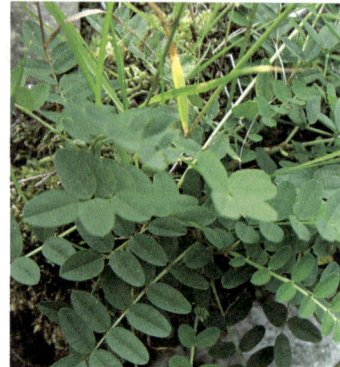

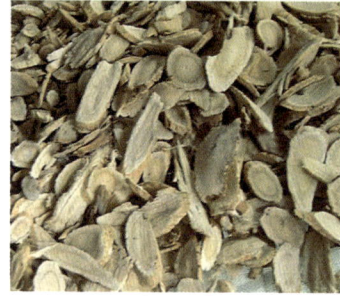

Astragalus

therapy. But it also has strong gastrointestinal side-effects (anorexia, nausea, vomiting, abdominal discomfort, diarrhea).

This is not meant to say that biomedicine does not have its merits. Many drugs produced by modern science do wonderful things with very few side-effects, especially if their dosage is low and administration period is short enough. Indeed, many patients are suggested to con-

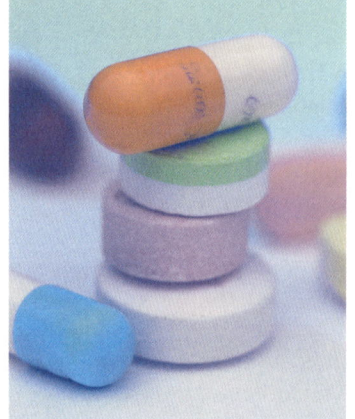

tinue care under a biomedical doctor even while getting treatment with Chinese medicine. But not attempting to restore the body's innate ability to maintain itself is contrary to the fundamental principles behind Chinese medicine.

Great importance is given to the concept behind the cliche, "Use it or lose it". The analogy we wish to draw from this is that the use of drugs that substitute for a function or substance will help relieve symptoms in the short term, but will lead to a decrease of function in the long run.

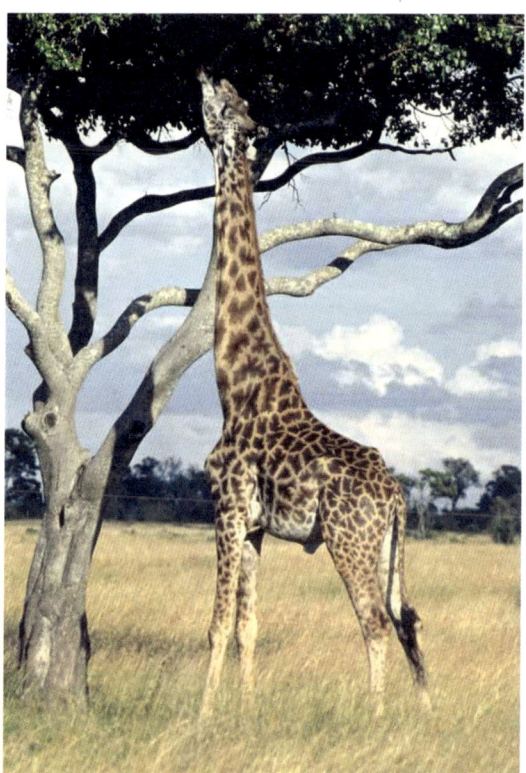

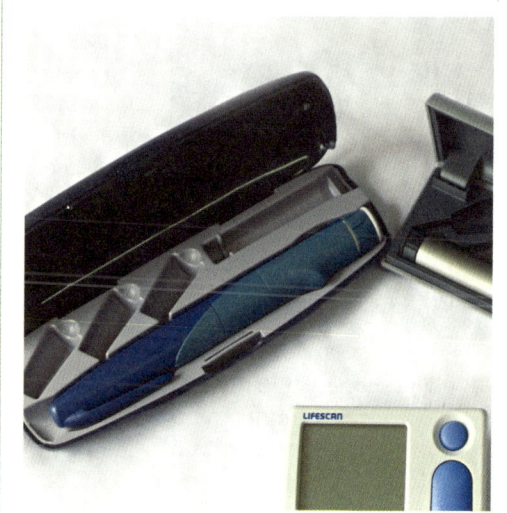

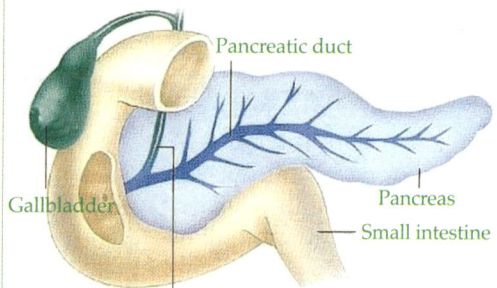

Insulin is essential to maintain blood sugar levels. But don't forget that once you begin to substitute for the substance produced by the body, the longer you use the synthetic substance, the less able your body will be to make it by itself. This type of treatment is inherently incomplete.

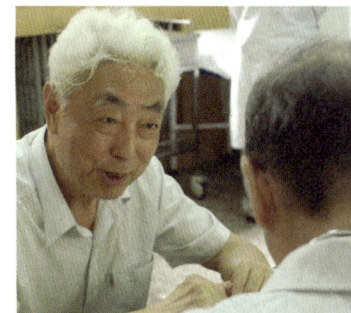

Chinese medicine focuses on treating the person, who happens to be ill; rather than concentrating on the disease mechanism, which happens to be inside a person like is done in biomedicine. The treatment methods of Chinese medicine, like other natural medical systems, are not intended to substitute for a bodily function or substance. They are intended to help the body do its job until it can do it itself.

As an example, modern research has shown that none of the common herbs used to manage infections can be compared to the potent antibiotics used in hospitals. Many of these herbs can only inhibit the bacteria, not destroy them. Yet experienced doctors of Chinese medicine will tell you that when properly prescribed, these herbs work well in treating infectious diseases. The supervisor of my master's degree clinical study, Professor Zhou Ping-an, who has worked in the hospital for over 40 years using Chinese medicine, is one of them. Often, Professor Zhou's use of Chinese medicine to manage infectious diseases is often more effective than biomedical treatment.

The underlying mechanism of the treatment methods used is to help the body recover using natural substances and manual methods to stimulate the body's general function. Eventually, when the body has been "re-trained" to maintain balance on its own, treatment can be reduced and then eliminated. The language it uses, qi, yin-yang, five phases, etc., is antique, but the idea it embraces is very advanced.

If you are ready to take an active role in your health care and in your life, Chinese medicine is right for you.

But remember, achieving good health is not like climbing a mountain, with a visible goal, but like maintaining a garden, giving constant care and paying attention to changes in the environment. Chinese medicine has been helping make what is sometimes seen as an arduous task a rewarding joy for millions of people for thousands of years. If you also want your garden to thrive, come and join the community of natural medicine, learn more about Chinese medicine.

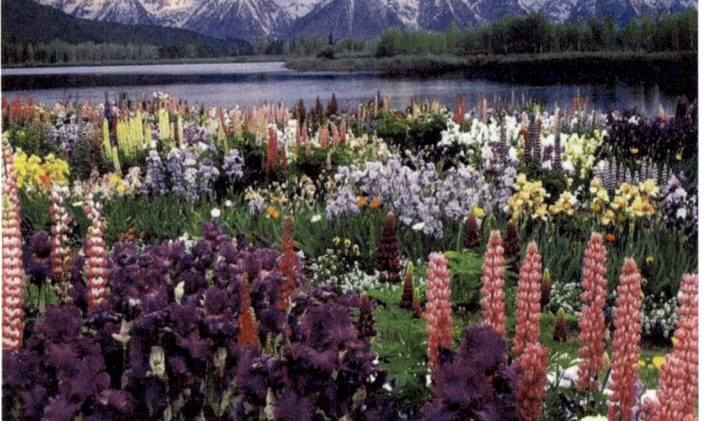

> Let us start by reading about a real case before introducing the basic concepts of Chinese medicine.

Case 1

Mr. Yu, 58, had suffered from hypertension and psychological problems for many years and presently complained of frequent dizziness, irritability, and insomnia. Four months before seeking treatment by Chinese medicine, his urine tested positive for glucose and his blood sugar level was higher than normal. He also reported needing to drink large amounts of fluid and excessive urination. He was diagnosed with type II diabetes mellitus and put on medication. After taking tolbutamide for a while, he still felt terrible, so he went to see Dr. Zhu Shi-mo for treatment with Chinese medicine. After taking a detailed history, inspecting his condition (general appearance, complexion, tongue), and taking his pulse, Dr. Zhu diagnosed him as having a weakness of the yin aspect of the kidney organ (these terms will be explained in detail in the coming chapters). The weakened yin and the internal heat accounted for all of Mr. Yu's major complaints. Dr. Zhu gave Mr. Yu an herbal prescription and told him to take it every day.

After taking the herbs for three weeks, he felt much better and his blood pressure was reduced. Another three weeks of treatment and the glucose in his urine disappeared and his blood sugar was coming down to normal levels. The medication necessary to treat his diabetes was gradually reduced and eventually stopped. In follow up visits, he remained healthy and lab results continued to be normal.

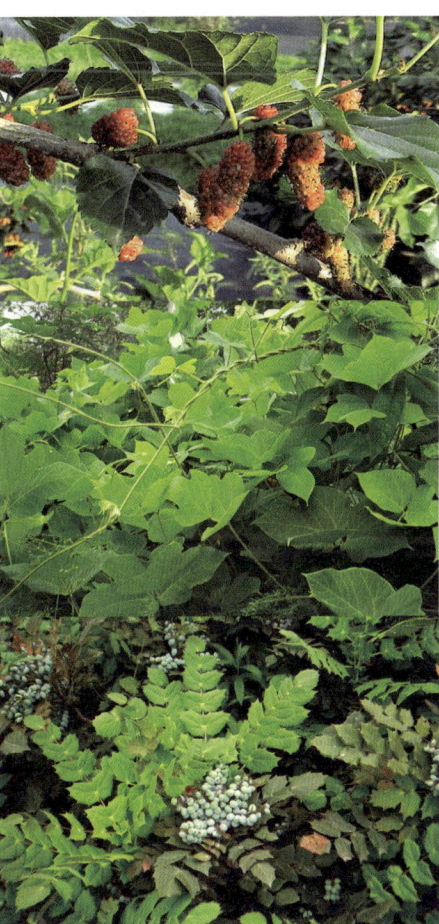

*All the cases in this book are from clinician's accounts, journal reports, or published books.

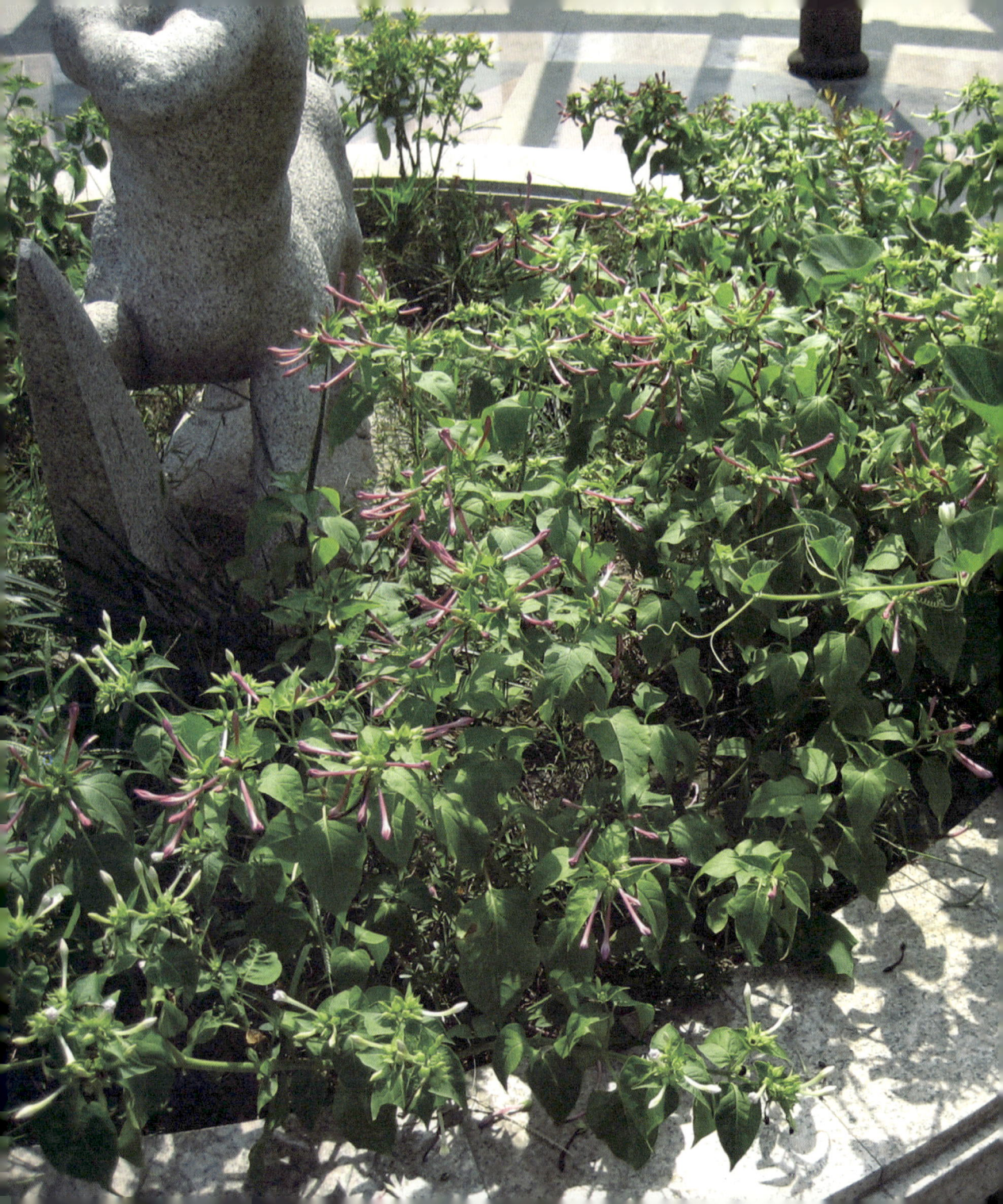

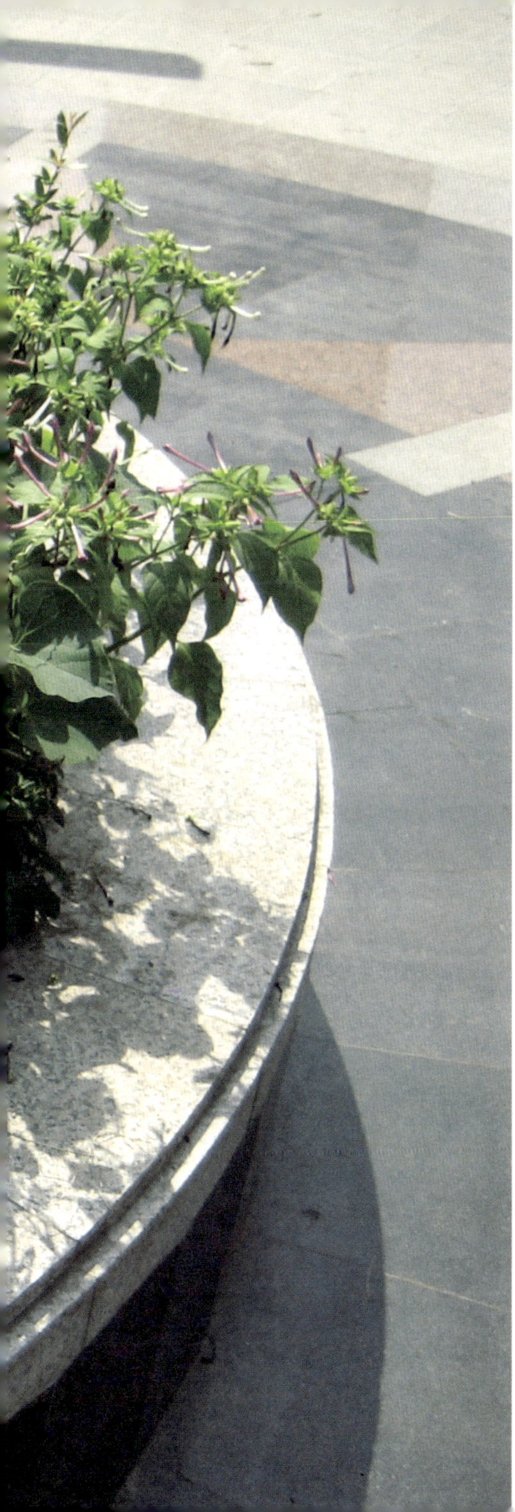

Chapter 2

How Does Chinese Medicine Understand Diabetes Mellitus?

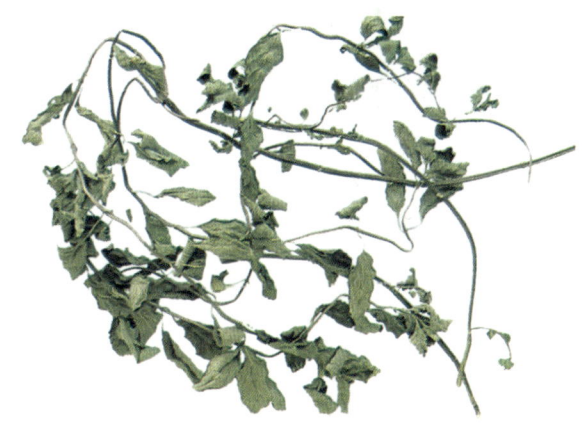

Many people in western countries are under the impression that Chinese medicine and acupuncture involve some kind of sorcery with needles or mysterious spirits. And indeed the ancient language of Chinese medicine can reinforce this view by referring to the "spirits" of the heart, lungs, liver, etc., or by insisting on the existence of the *jingluo*, which is the network that runs throughout the human body and is responsible for transporting qi and blood. However, to wise doctors and open-minded patients, the words used matter little, what is important is if the underlying concepts are able to be applied and beneficial results obtained.

Introduction to Chinese Medicine

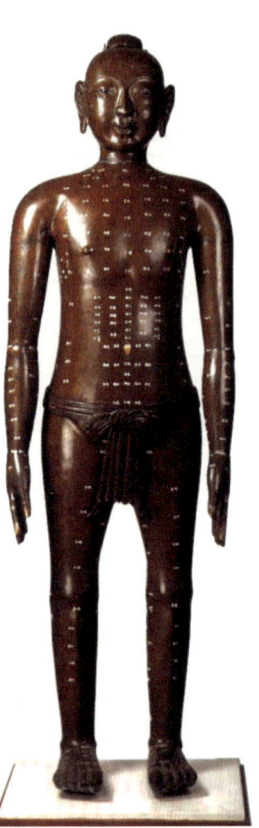

Chinese medicine enjoys a rich tradition and the longest continuous history among the world's natural medicines. Its legends suggest a history of 5000 years, while archeological evidence dates back to 1700 BC. The earliest existing literature dates from 200 BC and includes material from even earlier times. Chinese medicine is remarkable in having not only survived, but thrived during thousands of years of political and social ups-and-downs, and in remaining relevant and continuing to grow despite the rise of biomedicine. It is presently providing safe and effective care at an increasing rate to people all over the globe.

Perhaps an illustrative example of how Chinese medicine has greatly benefited society at large will help you understand its

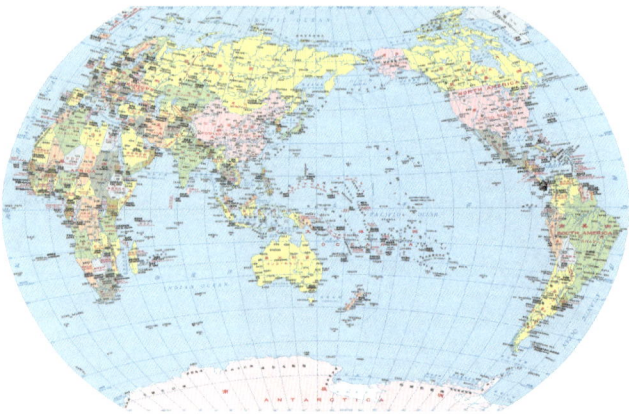

potential value to the world. During the infamous flu epidemic of 1918 that swept over the world causing millions of deaths, the death rate in China was reported lower than in other countries. It is estimated that over 2% of the world's population died during the flu with some countries suffering as much as a 20% loss of life. The statistics on China's southern province of Guangdong, however, say only 0.1% of the population died. During this time biomedical treatment was largely unavailable to the vast majority of China's huge population. The people relied on the methods and theories of Chinese medicine to maintain health and manage disease. It is incredible to think that this natural system of health care was effective against one of the deadliest, most rapidly spreading diseases in the past century.

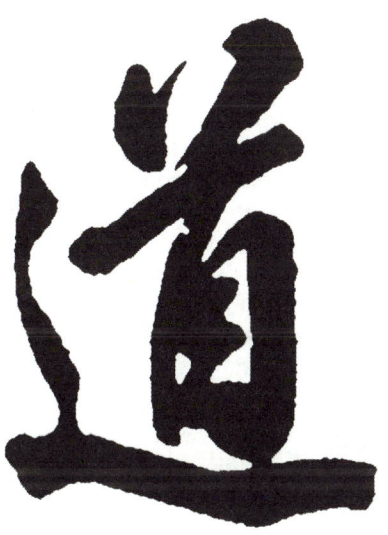

Dao

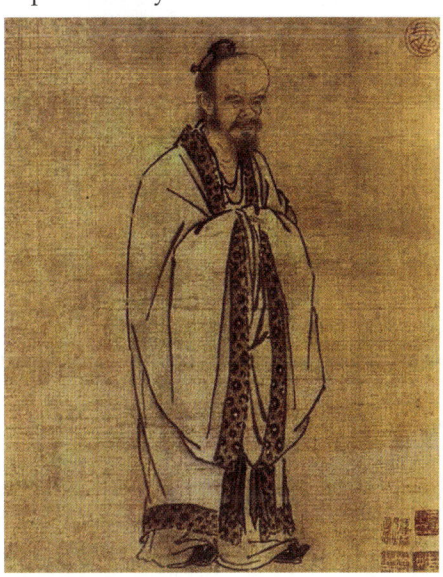

Lao Zi

Chinese medicine is based on the traditional philosophy and culture of ancient China, the essence of which is the relationship between man, the universe, and the Dao ("law" or "way") of nature. The Dao of nature is a dynamic relationship between yin and yang and health is the balance between yin and yang, as well as qi and blood within the body; and between the body and the external environment. When this balance is disrupted, disease, pain, and suffering arise. The basic principle of treatment in Chinese medicine is to discover and act on the fundamental cause of the imbalance to restore harmony to yin, yang, qi and blood, i.e. the ability of the body to heal itself.

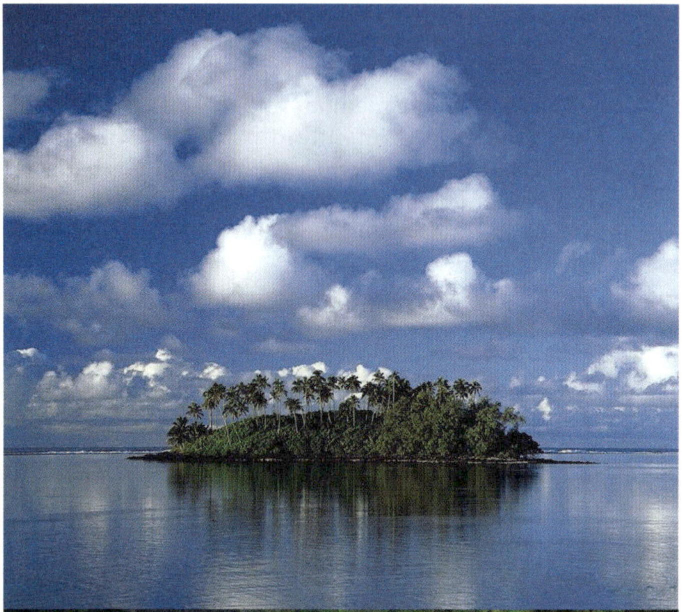

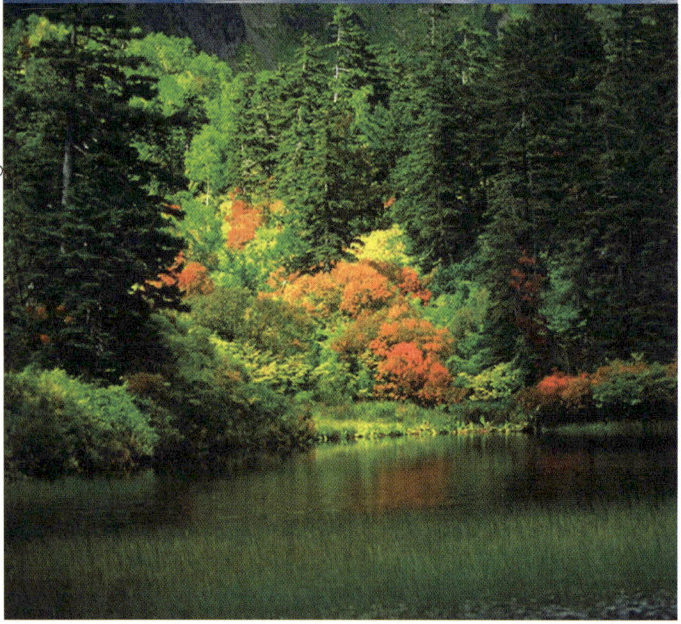

A famous patient

The famous Chinese legal figure Xie Jue-zai was diagnosed with diabetes in his sixties. He had all the typical symptoms: a strong thirst, frequent urination, and a dry mouth that was worse at night. He received biomedical treatment, modified his diet, and used single ginseng as well. But none of these treatments helped much with the symptoms. He decided to try Chinese medicine and was given Yu Quan San (Jade Spring Powder), a famous formula. After taking this powder for a while his symptoms disappeared. He was so pleased with the result he wrote a poem about it:

> This scholar's garden had thirsted for years, seeking an end to drought a spring was found!
> Firmly fasting or gobbling ginseng I tried them all.
> This little pill I came across ended up doing the trick.

Chinese medicine is as deep as an ocean, as wide as the sky, and can seem as complex as a jungle, but it is fundamentally a natural and simple system. Everything it encompasses can be understood in terms of yin, yang, and qi. For those who approach Chinese medicine from afar, the story begins with qi.

Two Key Concepts in Chinese Medicine

1. Qi

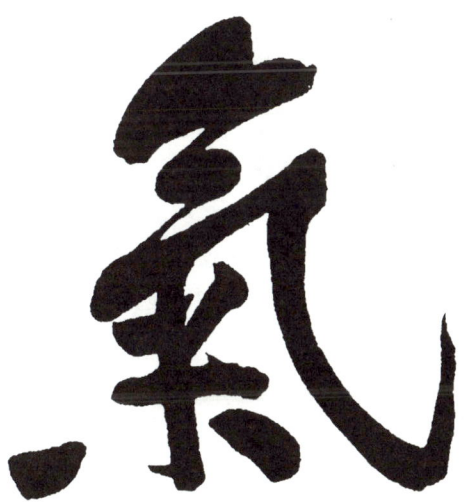

Qi (Chi)

The concept of qi is more than a medical term. Indeed, it is inseparable from ancient Chinese philosophy and is used by both fields to explain the forces that animate and control everything in the universe, from the cycle of seasons, to the origins and effects of emotions, to the inner workings of the human body. There is no simple literal English translation of qi. Different translators have rendered it as air, vapour, or energy and all of these are partially, but not completely, accurate.

The concept of qi is somewhat similar to "Pneuma" in ancient Greece or "Prana" in India, which were used to describe an underlying life force that was seen as having a strong connection to air and breath. Some of qi's important characteristics are:

- Qi is a kind of life force, but it is also a tangible vital substance that makes up everything in the cosmos, including human.
- Qi is the medium for transformation that stimulates the process of change. Everything in the universe, organic or inorganic, is made of qi and defined by qi. Mountains, rivers, animals, plants, even human emotions all have qi.
- Qi cannot be defined as simply "energy", nor can it be labeled a mere material substance, nor is it something in between. It is what connects humankind and the natural environment.
- Qi is the medium that makes the relationships and interactions between things and lives possible.

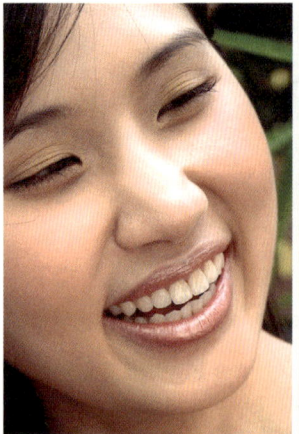
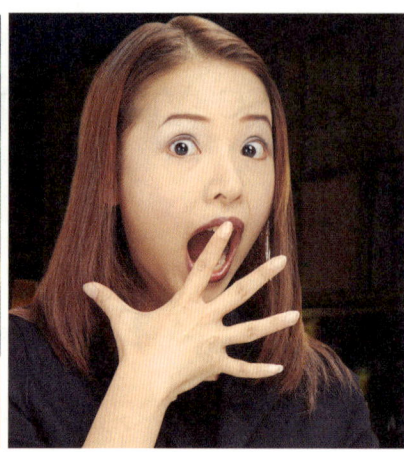

It can be difficult to understand the ancient Chinese claim that qi is both an ethereal life force as well as a material substance. To understand better, let us look at two very different categories of phenomena, human emotions and simple writing utensils, and see how qi exists in both of them.

First, take emotions. If a doctor of Chinese medicine was asked to describe the qi of the emotion of joy, he or she would probably say that its qi was light, rising, dispersing or possibly warm. On the other hand, if asked to describe the qi of fear, the words used would be more along the lines of dark, sinking, or cold. These descriptions are not based on any lab tests or scientific evidence, but are based primarily on the practitioner's own experience of the resonance between the emotional state and his or her perception.

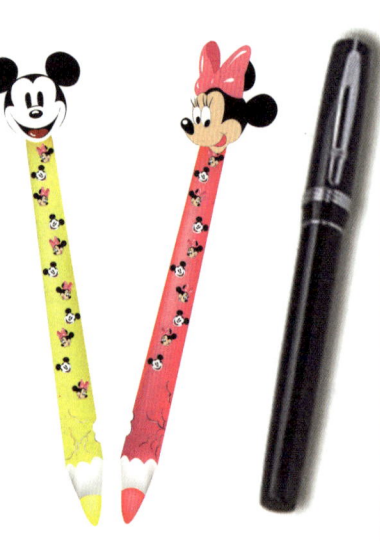

Now let us look at the other end of the spectrum, at two examples of solid, tangible writing utensils. One is a well-worn wooden pencil with teeth-marks and a Mickey Mouse design, the kind a first grader might use to scratch out the ABC's; the other is a sleek, expensive ink pen, probably black or silver that could be used to sign legal contracts. Similar to the description of joy above, the qi of the pencil could be described as light, familiar, or warm; and similar to the qi of fear above, the pen's qi would be described as dark, heavy, and cold. We can see that qi is not merely energy, as the physical substance of the pencils was a crucial part of describing their qi. Likewise, we see that qi cannot be limited to physical characteristics because the emotions described above, which have their distinct qi, have no tangible substance.

Chinese medicine, over thousands of years and with the help of countless doctors, patients, and philosophers has established a system in which the different phenomena of the universe can be described by qi and likewise the relationships between these phenomena can be described. Thus a Chinese doctor, when asked to describe the qi of something or the other, is not merely relying on his own experience and perceptions, but is using established theories to come up with an accurate description that anyone trained in qi will be able to agree with. In fact, it does not necessarily take training to understand qi. Most people would find the metaphorical descriptions of joy, fear, the pencil, and the pen easy to relate to. All people can think and talk in terms of qi, since it is based on the common sense of the natural world. The genius of Chinese medicine lies in its clear definitions and natural categorizations.

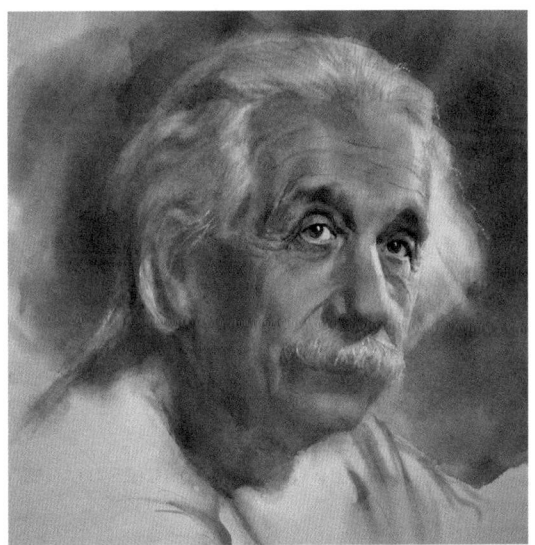
Albert Einstein

To understand what doctors of Chinese medicine aim to do in their treatments, we have to understand this well-used but rarely understood word, qi. Matter and energy are not independent of each other. As shown in the famous equation of Albert Einstein, $E=mc^2$, there is an intrinsic relationship between matter and energy. Qi is a concept of both matter and energy. It is the force that animates life. It is also the matter that constitutes life. Qi is shared by everything in the universe. It is the medium by which everything interacts. To quote one of the original textbooks of Chinese medicine in English:

"The interaction, or resonance, is realized by qi. Health is the harmonious resonance while disease is the disharmony. Components of the universe, the qi of herbs (plants, animal parts, and stones), acupuncture points (junctions of the human networks), lifestyle activities (movement and rest, food and relationships) or living environments (seasons, weather, or even air condition) share a resonating frequency that already exists in a person. A medicine or a conscious shift in a person's behavior can resonate with the condition within a person (e.g. a pattern of a disharmony) and induce a person toward health".

In terms of the human body and its various activities, Chinese medicine describes qi as having six major functions. They are as follows.

(1) Promoting: "Qi is the source of all movements".

Qi is a powerful substance that ignites and promotes all movements. Here "movement" is in its broadest sense and includes all physiological and psychological activities: walking, dancing, breathing, the heart beating, the blood flowing, the distribution of body fluids, speaking, thinking, birth, growth, development, maturation, and ageing. Qi promotes all normal functions of the human body.

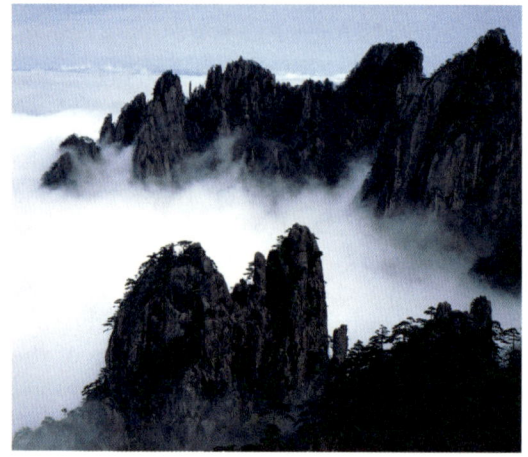

(2) Warming: "Qi warms the body and is the source of the heat energy of the body".

Maintenance of normal body temperature relies on the warming function of qi. This warming function also helps to smooth the flow and distribution of blood and body fluids. This warmth is also necessary for the internal organs to maintain normal function. The warmth can be manifested as the actual body temperature, in the normal function of the organs, or as the patient's subjective feeling of hot or cold. The difference between one person's qi and another's can partly explain why some people tend to wear more clothes than others even though the temperature is the same. When qi is deficient, internal cold might arise. When qi is excessive or accumulated, heat might appear.

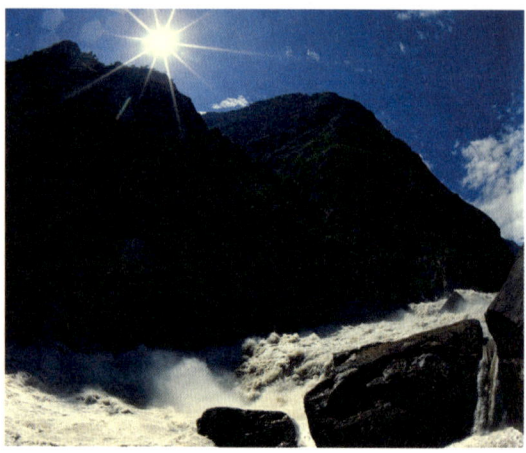

(3) Defending: "Qi protects the body, resisting the invasion of various external pathogens and preventing disease".

This function is often compared to immunity in biomedicine. Harmony of qi in the body is what protects us from pathogens in our environment. A quote from the most famous text of Chinese medicine, the *Yellow Emperor's Classic of Internal Medicine (Huáng Dì Nèi Jīng)* states: "If things from outside are able to harm the body, the qi must be weak." When qi is weak, we are vulnerable to disease. When qi is plentiful, we are less susceptible to illness. Qi can also help fight pathogens when they attack. The prognosis of disease is dependent on the dynamic balance sheet between the body's healthy qi and the attacking qi of the pathogenic factors.

(4) Securing: "Qi keeps things in their proper place".

This means controlling bodily substances such

as blood, urine, mucus, and saliva and preventing them from leaking out. It also describes the maintenance of the structural integrity of the body, helping to keep organs in their proper places. When this function is disrupted it will lead to problems such as bleeding or excessive secretion of body fluids, i.e. excessive sweating upon slight exertion, frequent urination, heavy bleeding during menstruation, or even organ proplapses or body parts like uterine or anal prolapse.

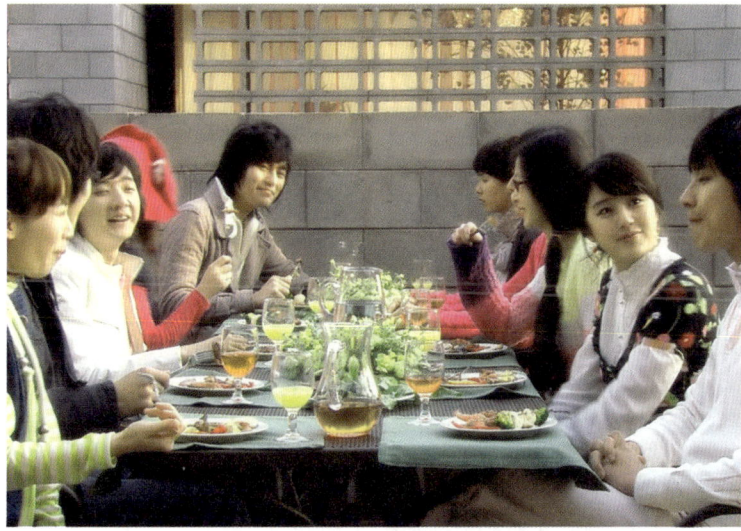

(5) Qi-transforming: "Qi is the source of transformation".

Changes in the body and mind are ascribed to the transformative function of qi. This can be compared to metabolism in biomedical terminology. For example, food is ingested and transformed into bodily substances. Emotional stress may influence the body and cause problems like headaches. For better or worse, these transformations are dependent on qi. Too much, too little, or improperly moving qi can cause different kinds of problems with the transformations that are managed by qi.

(6) Nurturing: "Qi of food and drink nourishes the body".

Qi is necessary for life, and its ability to give nutrition to the body comes mainly from the food we eat. Each food has its own particular qi and during digestion the food is transformed, the qi extracted and combined with body fluids. This then becomes blood and provides nutrition to the whole body. Chinese medicine calls this kind of qi "nutritive qi".

In summary, qi is the general force that animates the body's functions. Qi is also the material basis on which different parts of the body can interact. When our qi is healthy and plentiful, we enjoy physical and emotional well-being. This healthy qi can be easily disrupted if we don't take constant care. These disruptions can be caused by sudden weather changes, stress, unhealthy diet, or lack of proper physical activity.

The qi of diabetic patients is often disturbed and deficient. The following graph outlines some qi disorders of diabetic patients:

Table 2-1 Qi Disorders of Diabetic Patients

	Failure to promote	Failure to warm	Failure to defend	Failure to secure	Failure to transform	Fairlure to nuture
Pathological changes	Pancreas function impaired	May not be very common in diabetes, because it typically involves too much heat. At more severe stages cold symptoms may appear.	Susceptible to infection and common diseases like the common cold	Sugar coming out in the urine	Decreased production of insulin	Undernourished skin and eyes
Symptoms and signs	Weight loss; Fatigue; Weakness		Unhealing ulcers, easy infections	Frequent urination; Diarrhea	Weight loss despite increased food intake	Chapped and itching skin; Blurred vision

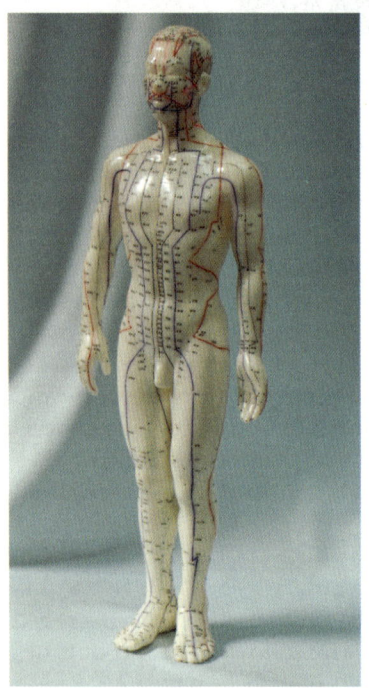

Channels on the Front

The basis of physiology, pathology, diagnosis, and treatment in Chinese medicine is the theory of essential qi. This theory's main principle is that essential qi is the basic substance that makes up the body. The physiological and pathological changes of the body are the results of normal and abnormal movements of qi respectively. Analyzing the movements of qi is an important part of diagnosis in Chinese medicine, Therefore, the purpose of treatment is to adjust these abnormalities of qi.

For example, some diabetes patients suffer from fatigue, shortness of breath, or sweating on the slightest exertion. Chinese medicine sees these symptoms as being caused by a weakness of qi while biomedicine fails to offer a satisfactory explanation. Fatigue and shortness of breath are because weak qi cannot support proper function and movement. The excessive sweating is due to qi not being able to keep the body's pores properly closed. By using herbs that supplement qi, like ginseng (*rén shēn*) or astragalus (*huáng qí*), these symptoms can be relieved,

Ginseng

and normal function restored. Modern research has revealed that these herbs contain effective active ingredients. For example, panaxoside in ginseng and both saponin and astragalus-polysaccharides in astragalus have been shown to boost immunity and relieve fatigue. This partially explains why the herbs work in clinic. But more research is needed to explain the larger picture of herbal medicine.

The meaning of qi is many faceted. Qi is what links man and nature, it is the material basis for all things. Chinese medicine has discovered that the qi of the internal organs can be reflected on the external parts of the body. The qi of the heart is manifested on the tongue, the qi of the liver is manifested in the eyes, the qi of the spleen (pancreas) can be seen on the mouth, while the qi of the lungs is evident on the nose, and the qi of the kidney can be observed on the ears. By observing the external manifestations, the functions of the internal organs can be inferred. Meanwhile, stimulus received externally can be conducted into the internal organs by qi. Acupuncture, moxibustion and massage are all based on the concept that qi in the channels can act on the internal organs.

These internal organ-sense organ correspondences may sound strange to many readers. Please remember that the Chinese understanding of the functions organs perform is different from the understanding of modern biomedicine. The organs in Chinese medicine are more than the anatomical structures seen separately in biomedicine. The Chinese understanding is based not only on the actual physical object, but on functions that relate to the system. The organ which is commonly translated as "spleen" in English actually performs the functions of the pancreas as well and is a central organ of digestion in Chinese medicine.

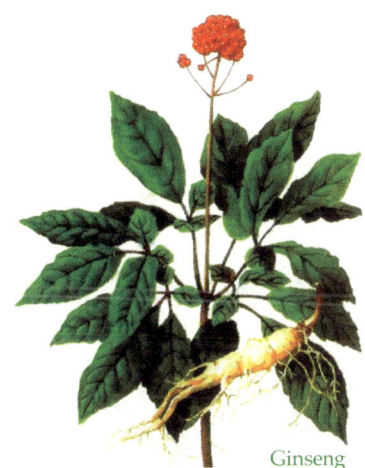

Ginseng

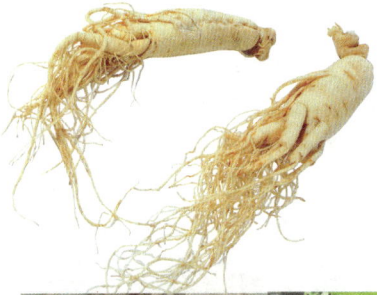

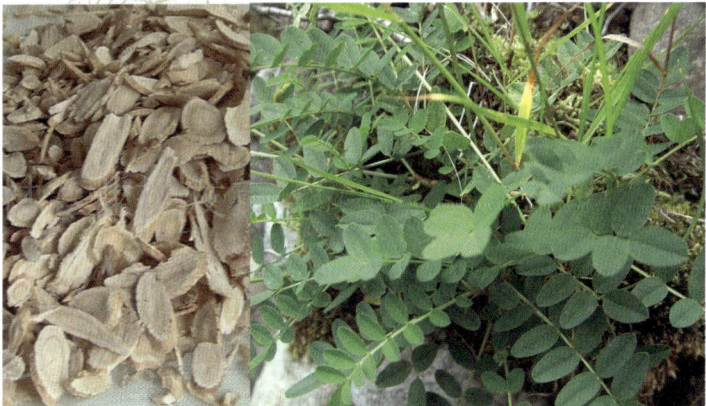

Astragalus

It is the fundamental, simple concepts that are most important and often neglected in learning. The idea of qi, along with yin-yang theory, is of utmost importance to Chinese medicine. Without qi, there is death; with qi, there is life. Try not to form a fixed idea about what qi is after this short explanation. Keep an open mind and deepen your understanding of qi as we explore more about Chinese medicine.

Case 2

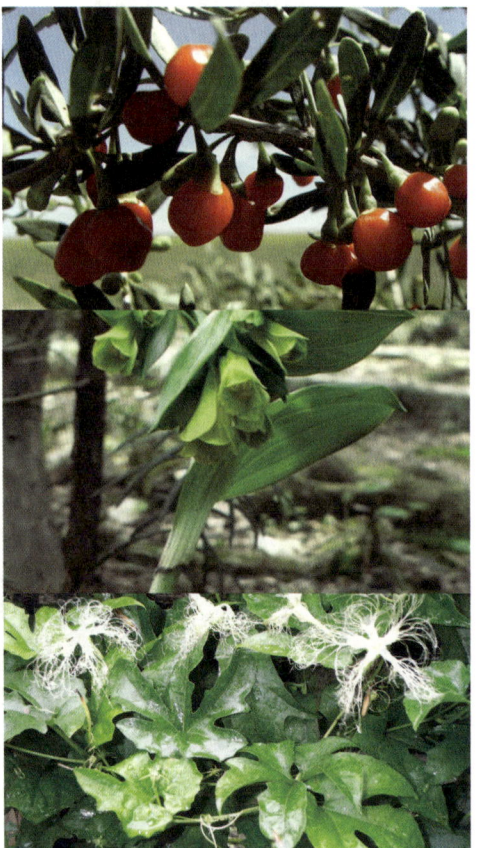

Mr. Gu had been suffering from diabetes for years. He had all the typical symptoms including thirst, excessive drinking, an increased appetite, and frequent, cloudy urination. Most of all, he complained of severe fatigue and weakness aggravated by the slightest exertion. He decided to see Dr. Shi Jinmo for treatment with Chinese medicine. Dr. Shi diagnosed him as having a deficiency of both qi and yin. Since the patient's most severe symptoms were fatigue and weakness, priority was given to supplementing qi. Mr. Gu's qi was not strong enough to maintain his energy throughout the day or to give his muscles enough strength.

The formula prescribed used large dosages of ginseng and astragalus, which are major herbs for boosting qi. After taking just a week's worth of herbs, Mr. Gu felt much better. Seeing that his qi had recovered a little bit, Dr. Shi changed the prescription to supplement qi and yin at the same time. Gradually, over the next several weeks his blood sugar was brought down to normal levels. In addition, the symptoms that were bothering him disappeared completely. Very pleased with the results, Mr. Gu has stopped regular treatment, but will continue to take a small dose of herbs in pill form to consolidate the effect of treatment.

2. Yin-yang

Originally, the words yin and yang were used to describe the sides of a mountain that predominately faced away or towards the sun respectively. In other words, the side facing the sun pertains to yang while the side facing away from the sun is yin.

Due to the regular rotation of the earth, each individual mountain will have one side that mostly faces the sun, which is the yang side, and one side that usually faces away from the sun, which is the yin side. Indeed because of the regular change from darkness to light due to the rotation of the earth, everything has an intrinsic yin aspect and yang aspect. The rotation of our planet has caused everything on it to evolve in such a way that it adapts to the cyclic coming of light and dark. Yin and yang are inseparable characteristics of being a part of planet Earth.

The concept of unified duality is key to ancient Chinese culture, and the Chinese understanding of every natural and social phenomena is based on this. There are always two (with a relationship), not an isolated one. Harmony is the balance between the two. Later on, this concept of unified duality was extended to embrace all phenomena on the planet and in the universe.

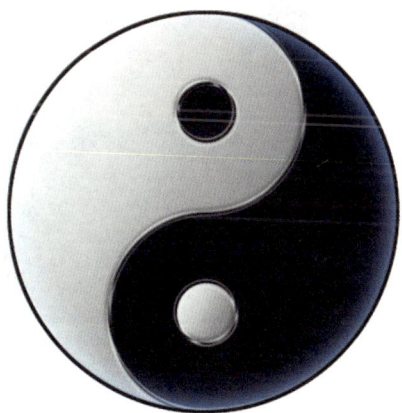

Figure 2-1 Yin-yang of Tai Ji

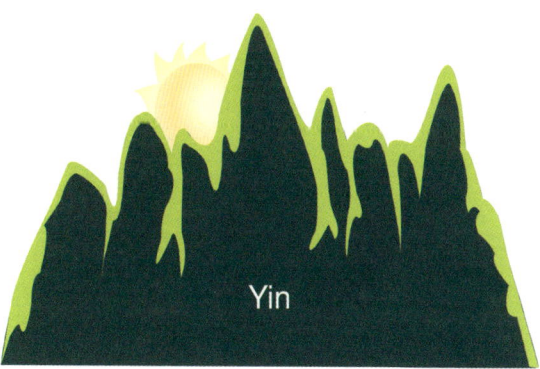

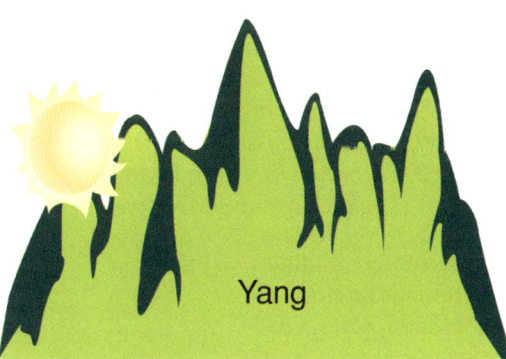

Yang is associated with such qualities such as brightness and warmth while yin is associated with the opposing characteristics of darkness and cold. Some further examples are: daytime pertains to yang while night is yin; sunny weather is yang while cloudy weather is yin; spring and summer are yang and autumn and winter are yin; fire is yang while water is yin, and so on. Further expansion of this logic leads to the division of everything in the universe into yin or yang based on the quality, property, position, trend, function, or effect of the phenomena being classified.

The concept of yin-yang is the general division of any given thing (including living things, inanimate objects, feelings, actions, etc.) into two polar attributes which are related to each other. Yin and yang can also be used to subdivide already classified categories. For example, we already described summer as yang, but during summer there are days when it is extremely hot (more yang) and days when it is cloudy and cooler (more yin). In other words, yin-yang can be infinitely divided. The complementary and opposing nature of yin and yang can be used as labels to describe two opposing things or two opposing aspects contained within one thing. See the following table for a clearer picture of the categorization of yin and yang.

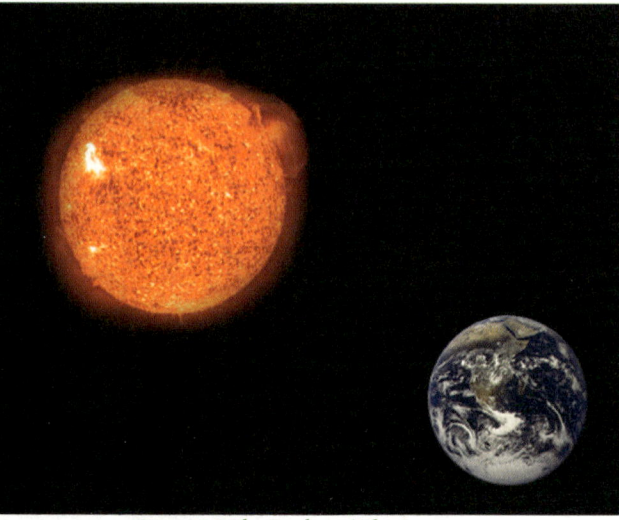

Figure 2-2 The Earth and The Sun

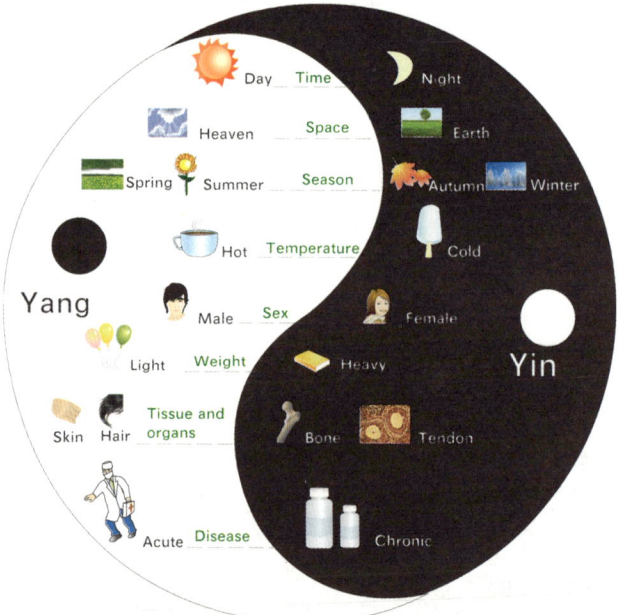

Figure 2-3 Examples of Yin-yang Categorization

Table 2-2 Categorization of Yin & Yang

Category	Yang	Yin
Time	Day	Night
Space	Heaven	Earth
Season	Spring, Summer	Autumn, Winter
Temperature	Hot	Cold
Weight	Light	Heavy
Speed	Fast	Slow
Motion	Up and out, Vigorous	Down and in, Subtle
Brightness	Light	Dark
Sex	Male	Female
Tissue and organs	Skin, Hair	Bone, Tendon
Disease	Acute	Chronic

In Chinese medicine the fundamental definition of health is when there is a good balance of yin and yang in the body. Diagnosis of disease and its treatment are all aimed at restoring this equilibrium. This may sound simplistic, but when you consider the fact that all of the organs, functions, emotions, fluids, and structures each have yin and yang aspects that must be balanced, you can see how the doctor's job of detecting every imbalance using no more than the five senses is a very difficult task.

Yin and yang are interdependent. This means that the condition of one will affect the other. If there is too little yin, then yang will appear to be in excess; and if there is too much yin, there will appear to be too little yang. The reverse is of course true for when there is too little or too much yang. A simple example can be seen when the body's temperature rises or falls too much. With fever there is a relative abundance of yang heat. This means the cool yin aspect of the body is not sufficient to counteract the heat. Therefore the practitioner must restore the balance of yin and yang by making the cool yin aspect of the body equal to the hot yang aspect. Likewise, if a patient has hypothermia and has dangerously low body temperature there is a relative abundance of yin cold in relation to yang heat.

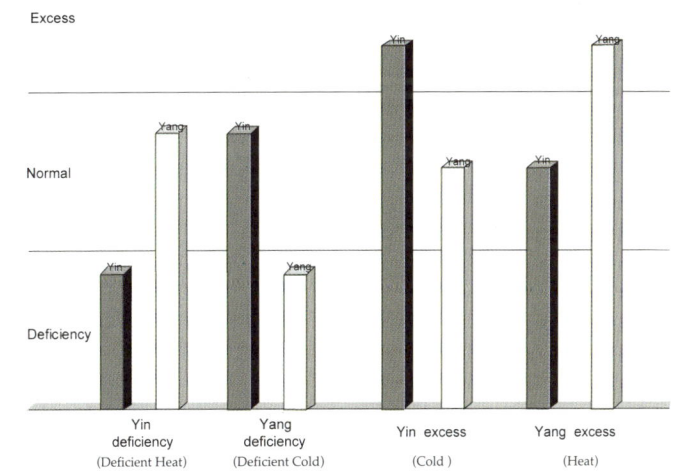

Figure 2-4 Ying-yang Disorders

*This is only a simplied model to help you understand. Remember: Yin and yang are always a pair.

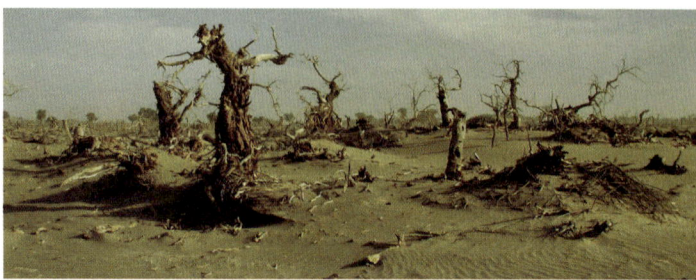

However, it is not enough to know merely which is the stronger of yin or yang and which is the weaker. If there is heat, for example, this could be due to either too much yang and yin being relatively weak, or it could be because there is not enough yin and therefore yang only appears to be in excess.

This is a difficult concept for all beginning students of Chinese medicine so let us look at an example. A forest that has not had any rain for many months will be dry and probably hot. Dryness and heat are yang qualities as opposed to yin moisture and cold. A forest that is on fire is also in a condition of yang heat. In each case, the yang aspect is greater than the yin aspect. But to restore the yin-yang balance of both situations, one must choose different strategies. To restore the forest in drought it is necessary to add yin, meaning water. On the other hand, to balance a blazing fire, one has no other option but to remove the excess yang fire. In Chinese medicine, the dry forest would be said to be in a state of yin deficiency, where the heat is due to a relative abundance of yang. The forest fire is a state of yang excess, where yin may very well be normal. The other states are yang deficiency and yin excess. Please see the diagrams to better understand the four different types of yin-yang imbalances.

A patient diagnosed with an excess of yang will have yang-type symptoms such as high fever, restlessness, red complexion, rapid pulse, or yellowish tongue coating since an excess of yang leads to heat. The heat of excess yang can damage the cool water of yin and can be seen when the patient has symptoms like dry mouth and throat, thirst, dry tongue.

Table 2-3 Manifestations of Yin-yang Disorders

	Typical Manifestations
Yang excess	Fever, aversion to heat, thirst, desire for cold drinks, reddish complexion, restlessness, yellowish-colored mucus, dark-colored urination, constipation, red tongue, yellowish tongue coating, rapid pulse
Yin excess	Aversion to cold, no thirst, desire for warm drinks, thin and watery mucus, loose stool, pale complexion, light-colored tongue, whitish tongue coating, slow or tense pulse
Yang deficiency	Preference for warmth, cold limbs, pale complexion, spontaneous sweating, fatigue, shortness of breath, loose stool, enlarged and light-colored tongue, whitish tongue coating, deep, slow and weak pulse
Yin deficiency	Thirst, dry mouth and throat, hot feeling in the soles and palms, afternoon fever, night sweating, red tongue with little coating, rapid and fine pulse

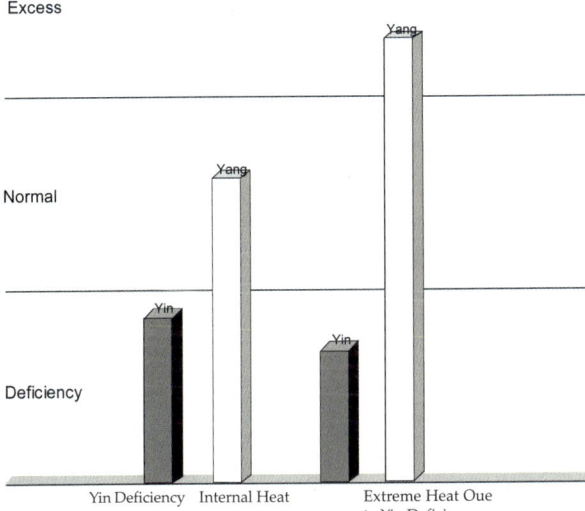

Figure 2-5 Deficient Heat

For diabetic patients, the typical pathogenesis in Chinese medical terms is yin deficiency leading to heat of a deficiency type. The typical symptoms "polydipsia, polyphagia, excessive urination and weight loss" are due to yin damage and deficient heat or fire. This deficient heat is not caused by excess of yang but relative abundance of yang in relation to the lack of yin. Of course, this diagnosis cannot apply to every patient, but it is the most common underlying mechanism.

A person may be born with a tendency to develop heat from yin deficiency or it might be acquired through life. Improper diet and disturbed emotions will disrupt qi flow. This stagnation will cause internal fire. To understand how stagnant qi produces fire, think of a traffic jam in a narrow tunnel. All those engines (qi) will start to heat the place up if they don't move. Fire will then consume qi (as a flame exhausts oxygen) as well as yin. So both qi and yin have been damaged. This is why diabetic patients tend to have a complex syndrome of both qi and yin deficiency with internal heat.

In clinic every patient may present with a different syndrome, or usually a combination of syndromes, because every patient is different. Even for one patient, depending on the development of the disease, life style modifications adopted, or environmental changes, the diagnosis will also have to be modified and refined at each specific stage.

The diagnosis of yin or yang is based on an integrative and insightful analysis of all the symptoms and signs of each individual patient.

After all of the information about a patient is collected, the data will be vigorously analyzed and categorized by an experienced practitioner into different patterns of disharmony. The patterns can be numerous, and will vary with the individual, time, location, climate and other factors involved. Corresponding treatment protocol will be made according to the specific patterns identified. Chinese medicine is aimed at highly individualized treatment — the goal of all types of medicine. Chinese medicine's goal is the recovery of the innate function of the body, a true medicine.

Note: Five element theory is also an important fundamental element of Chinese medicine. Yet for diabetes we have chosen to focus on qi and yin-yang. Please refer to other books in this series or to the suggested reading list for more information on this aspect of Chinese medicine.

Case 3

A patient named Mr. Wu, 68, who had suffered from diabetes for 10 years, came into the clinic seeking treatment with Chinese medicine in October of 2005. Having his blood sugar levels controlled with pharmaceuticals, his symptoms of thirst, frequent urination, and increased appetite were not that obvious. He mainly complained of edema in the lower legs, a need to urinate frequently at night, numbness and tingling in the toes, feeling cold with cold extremities, shortness of breath, weakness, lassitude, and soreness and weakness in the lower back and knees. On examination, his light-red tongue with teeth marks and a thin and whitish coating, and the deep, fine, and weak pulse indicated a bodily weakness. His biomedical doctors had diagnosed him with diabetic neuropathy.

In Chinese medicine the final pattern diagnosis was a deficiency of yin and yang complicated by the stagnation of qi and blood. Kidney yang's function in the body is to be the foundation of warmth, as well as ruling over body fluids especially in the lower body. When this yang is weakened and the warmth declines the patient will feel cold and his arms and legs will feel cold to the touch. When kidney yang's control of fluid metabolism is disrupted the need to urinate at night will increase (night is when yang is weakest) and fluid will accumulate causing edema. The other signs and symptoms are mainly related to the stagnation of qi and blood or the general weakness of the body's qi.

An herbal prescription that addressed all the patient's patterns was chosen and the patient was told to come back in a week. In just this short time Mr. Wu started feeling much better. He continued taking his Acarbose 50mg (three times a day) and Monopri l4mg (once a day), and eventually his lab results improved. He also had much more energy and his other symptoms were greatly relieved. Mr. Wu's case is a serious one and he continues to get support from both biomedicine and Chinese medicine.

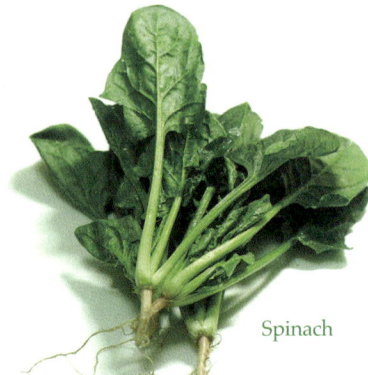
Spinach

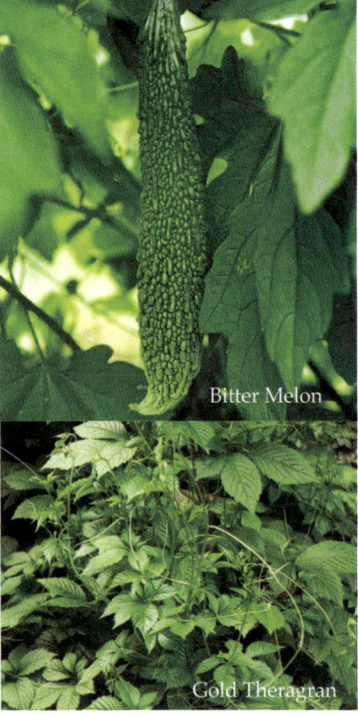
Bitter Melon

Gold Theragran

Diabetes Mellitus in Chinese Medicine

Diabetes was named by the British doctor Thomas Willis in 1672, and means "sweet urine". Chinese medicine recognized this disease as early as 400 BC in the *Yellow Emperor's Classic of Internal Medicine (Huáng Dì Nèi Jīng)* with descriptions of the typical symptoms of thirst, hunger and emaciation. Chinese doctors labeled this disease *"xiao ke"* which means "emaciation and thirst". This was the name used until the modern definition of diabetes was formed. In this text the causes of the diseases were attributed to innate constitution (those who have a weakness of the major internal organs are more susceptible to diabetes), diet (caused by food high in fat and calories) and emotions (anger causes qi to go upward, heat leads to emaciation).

Wang Tao, an official in the Tang dynasty (618-907) suggested tasting the patient's urine to help diagnose diabetes and monitor its progress. He also said that eating pig pancreas could treat diabetes. Wang Tao ascribed the cause of diabetes to kidney deficiency while Sun Si-miao (581-682), another famous doctor of the same period, attributed diabetes to dietary irregularities. Later Liu He-jian (1110-1200), a doctor in the Jin dynasty, emphasized the role of emotional disturbances.

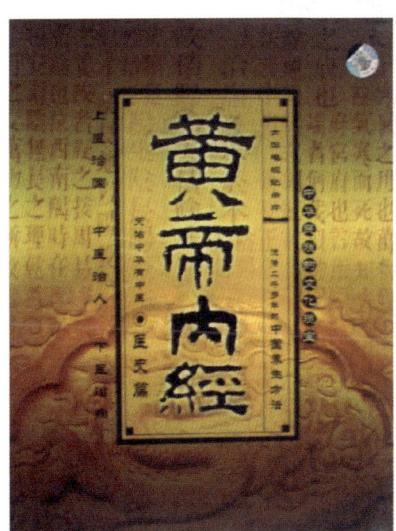

The Yellow Emperor's Classic of Internal Medicine (Huáng Dì Nèi Jīng)

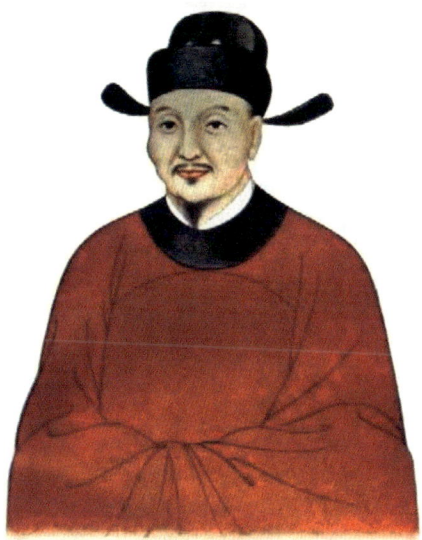

Wang Tao

Wang Tao quoted Zhen Li-yan from his *Records of Proven Formulas Past and Present* (*Gǔ Jīn Lù Yàn*, 627 A.D.) to summarize Chinese medicine's understanding of *xiao ke*:

There are three kinds of *xiao ke*. Thirst, excessive drinking, frequent and sweet (tasting) urine are characteristics of "*xiao ke*" (refers to the typical diabetes presentation). Thirst, excessive eating and oily (looking) urination are characteristics of "*xiao zhong*" (refers to chyluria, or the presence of fatty substances in the urine). The syndrome of thirst yet unable to drink, frequent urination, swollen legs, emaciation, and impotence are characteristics of "*shen xiao*" (describes the late stage of diabetes with complications).

This record from hundreds of years ago summarizes the characteristics of the whole process of diabetes.

Over the centuries, Chinese medicine's understanding of diabetes has been developing. As early as the Eastern Han dynasty of 25–220 A.D., Zhang Zhong-jing, one of Chinese medicine's most revered figures, had already established the standard pattern identification and basic formulas for *xiao ke*.

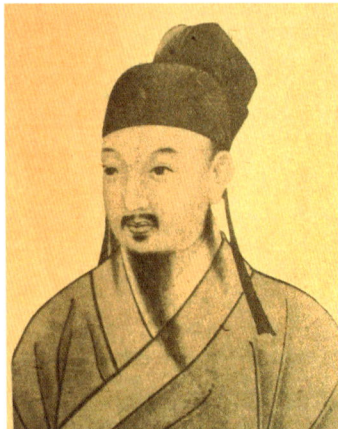

Zhang Zhong-jing

Ever since that, practitioners of Chinese medicine at different times have been contributing to the understanding and treatment of diabetes.

Chinese medical theory states that the fundamental mechanism of diabetes is internal heat due to yin deficiency. This internal heat is not excess heat resulting from an excess of yang. The heat is a manifestation of a relative abundance of yang due to yin deficiency. This yin deficiency may be constitutional, from a habitually unhealthy diet, from emotional disturbances, from external pathogens, or most often, from a combination of these risk factors.

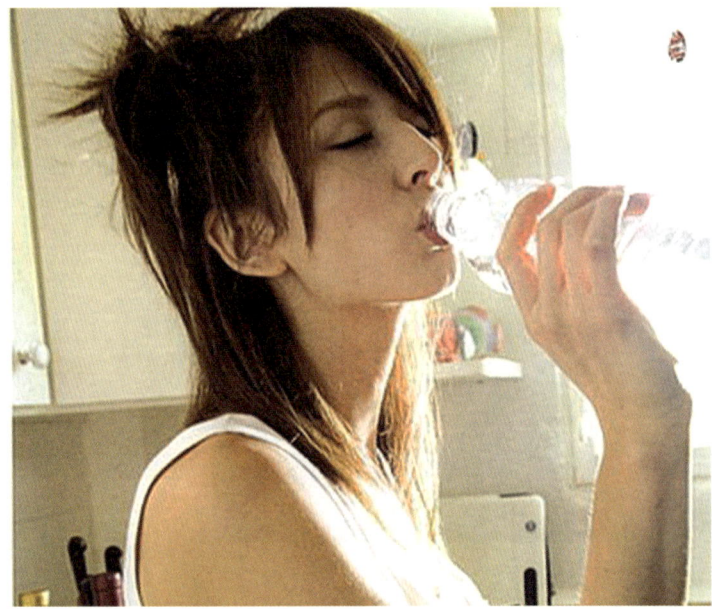

The presence of heat and the lack of fluids account for many of the common symptoms of diabetes. Excess thirst is obviously a condition of dryness and heat. And an increased appetite is seen as the stomach doing its job too fast, stimulated by heat. This heat can also consume the body's healthy qi leading to a deficiency of qi. This can cause the diabetic patient to feel weakness, fatigue and lassitude. The weakness of qi's defensive function can also explain why patients with diabetes are more vulnerable to infections. When there is any kind of imbalance in the body it will not stay isolated. A problem with qi will eventually affect blood, yin, yang, and other bodily substances and functions. When blood is affected, it might lead to blood deficiency or stagnation, and manifest as various complications involving the eyes, heart, kidney, and other organs. In the long run, yang will also be affected, resulting in deficiency of both yin and yang, and ultimately leading to death.

Yin deficiency and internal heat

First, internal heat arises from an inherent deficiency of yin and/or your diet, emotions, life style lead to the formation of heat as well as damage yin. This pathological heat will then consume yin fluids, gradually but steadily. More symptoms begin to present like a strong thirst, increased appetite, frequent urination, and decreasing weight. For some patients, these typical symptoms may not be prominent or even present at all because of another disturbance of qi which will cause other patterns to manifest predominately. Because many diabetics are overweight, there are often patterns involving excess dampness and phlegm*. Since Chinese medicine treats the whole patient, addressing predominant pathologies is given priority while still paying attention to protecting yin and cooling heat.

*Excess fat is often considered a form of dampness or phlegm in Chinese medicine which is the result of poor digestion and improper fluid metabolism, often related to qi disorders.

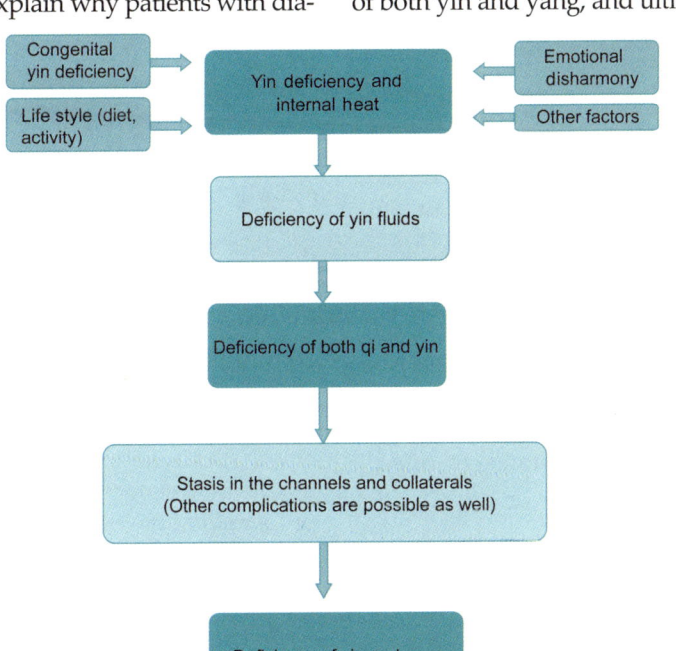

Figure 2-6 The Pathomechanism of Diabetes in Chinese Medicine

Chinese medical treatment gives priority to treatment based on pattern differentiation (*Biàn Zhèng Lùn Zhì*). This is the way that Chinese medicine categorizes, understands, and manages all types of illnesses. It is a highly individualized principle and is always integrated with the disease diagnosis.

So what is a pattern (*Zhèng*)?

A pattern, similar to the concept of syndrome, is a group of interrelated signs and symptoms that together reveal the fundamental characteristics of a patient's condition. Chinese medicine believes that manifestations (symptoms and signs) mirror the performance of internal organs. So a pattern is the reflection of an underlying pathomechanism, often called the root of the disease in Chinese medicine. Over thousands of years, Chinese medicine has accumulated a large amount of experience in summarizing and categorizing these patterns in the most innovative ways. It now uses them as the guidelines in prescribing treatment. Disease diagnosis and pattern diagnosis go together and guide the practitioner to the proper treatment. There is a saying in Chinese medicine, "Different diseases, same treatment; same disease, different treatment". This saying underscores the importance to individualized pattern diagnosis in Chinese medicine.

The patterns described below are some of the most typically seen in diabetes patients at various stages of disease development.

Deficiency of both yin fluids and qi

As explained above, yin and qi are often damaged in the diabetic patient. These deficiencies may present symptoms concurrently, or at different times. Qi deficiency may make you feel fatigued, lazy, and inactive. You may have less energy, low spirits, or even shortness of breath. Yin deficiency causes thirst and dry mouth, a feeling of heat in the afternoon, and irritability. Generally speaking, this pat-

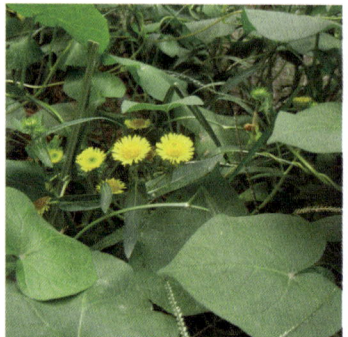

Table 2-4 Typical Symptoms of Qi Deficiency and Yin Deficiency

Qi deficiency	Yin deficiency
Weakness	Irritability
Fatigue on slight exertion	Thirst and dry mouth
Laziness, spiritlessness	A feeling of heat in the afternoon
Shortness of breath	A hot feeling in the palms and soles

tern is more serious than simple yin deficiency with some internal heat which was described above.

Blood stagnation and channel blockage

As diabetes progresses, blood will be affected. Qi is deficient and cannot promote proper blood flow. Stagnation of blood leads to many serious complications. There will be all kinds of vessel problems, affecting anywhere from the eyes to the feet, causing vision problems (diabetic retinopathy),

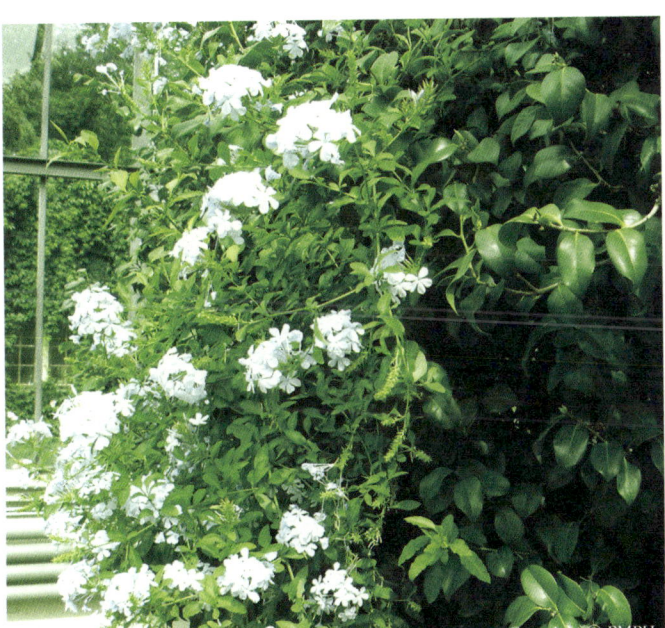
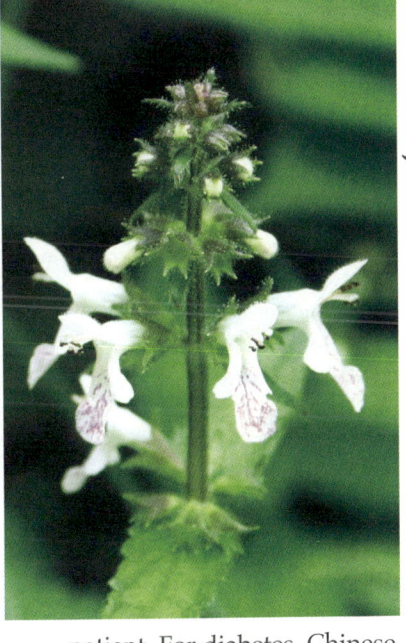

hardening of the arteries, skin problems, etc. Channels are the pathways of qi and blood. When blood is stagnated, the channels are blocked, causing numbness, tingling sensations, and eventual loss of function.

Deficiency of yin and yang

At the final stage, both yin and yang will be affected. Numerous serious problems are possible. The organs are seriously damaged. All kinds of complaints crop up and don't respond to treatments that worked at earlier stages.

This is simply the theoretical progression of diabetes in Chinese Medicine. Usually, your pattern will not be as simple as those listed above, it will often have multiple facets. The pattern of an individual patient is often mixed with other underlying conditions. This sequence isn't written in stone either. With early treatment and attention to lifestyle habits, the progression can be stopped or slowed.

The above is how Chinese medicine generally understands diabetes, not about a specific patient. For diabetes, Chinese medicine recognizes the key pathomechanism as yin deficiency and internal heat. Based on this understanding, the basic treatment methods all act to eliminate heat and supplement yin along with paying close attention to the individual characteristics of each patient.

Another important division of diabetes is based on the symptoms. Since the Tang and Song dynasties, *xiao ke* (emaciation and thirst-diabetes) has been divided into three types and treated respectively. They are:

> ### Upper *xiao*
> The main complaint is a strong thirst and dry mouth and tongue. This is due to heat in the lungs. Clearing lung heat is the major treatment method here.
>
> ### Middle *xiao*
> The main complaint is hunger and an increased food intake, emaciation, and dry stool. It is due to heat in the stomach. Here it is important to concentrate on clearing stomach heat.
>
> ### Lower *xiao*
> The main complaint is frequent and excessive urination or oily urination. It is due to deficient kidneys. Supplementing kidney yin is the priority in this case.

In clinic, diabetic patients often will encompass two or even three of the above categories. The point of this division is to highlight your major symptoms and the reason for them. The treatment will be slightly different for each category, even if they are all present at the same time. Upper *xiao* requires herbs that clear lung heat and moisturize lung yin; for middle *xiao* herbs that clear stomach heat are used. If all three *xiao* are present, practitioners will decide how to vary treatment according to the severity of the symptoms.

Biomedicine has provided modern Chinese medicine with a more detailed picture of diabetes. With the aids of modern technology, Chinese medicine is able to understand diabetes using both sophisticated philosophy and the latest technology. Pattern identification and evaluation of treatments become more precise with the ability to track blood sugar levels and the use of other lab tests. The latest guidelines for the treatment of diabetes with Chinese medicine to be issued soon will provide references on pattern identification, recommended treatment protocols, and treatment evaluation standards at every stage of the disease. The treatment of diabetes with Chinese medicine has been developing over thousands of years. Its methods and theories are not fixed or stagnant and will continue to develop over time.

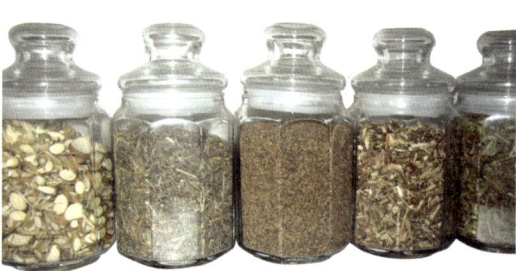

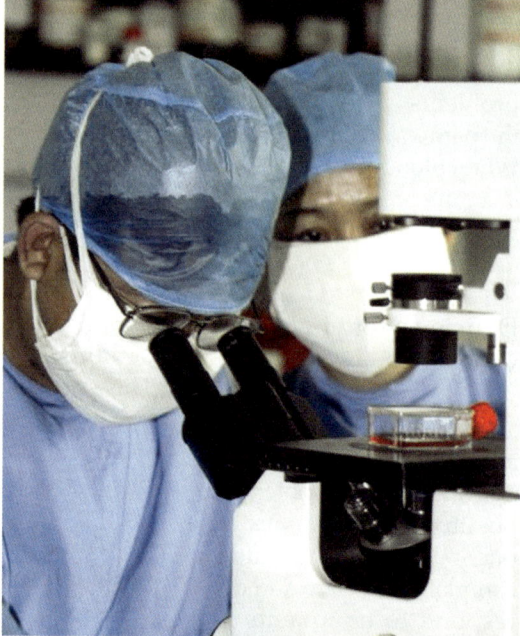

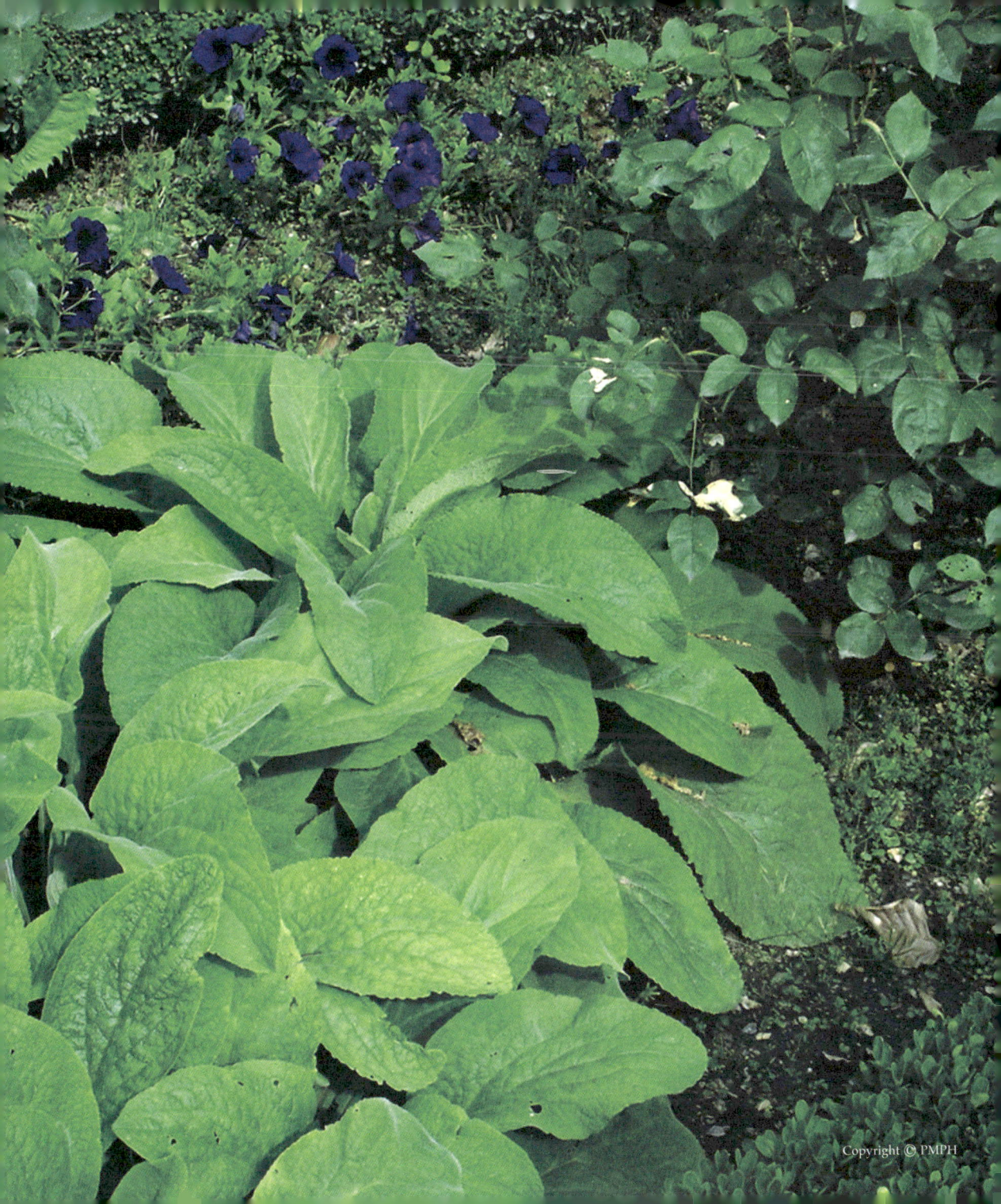

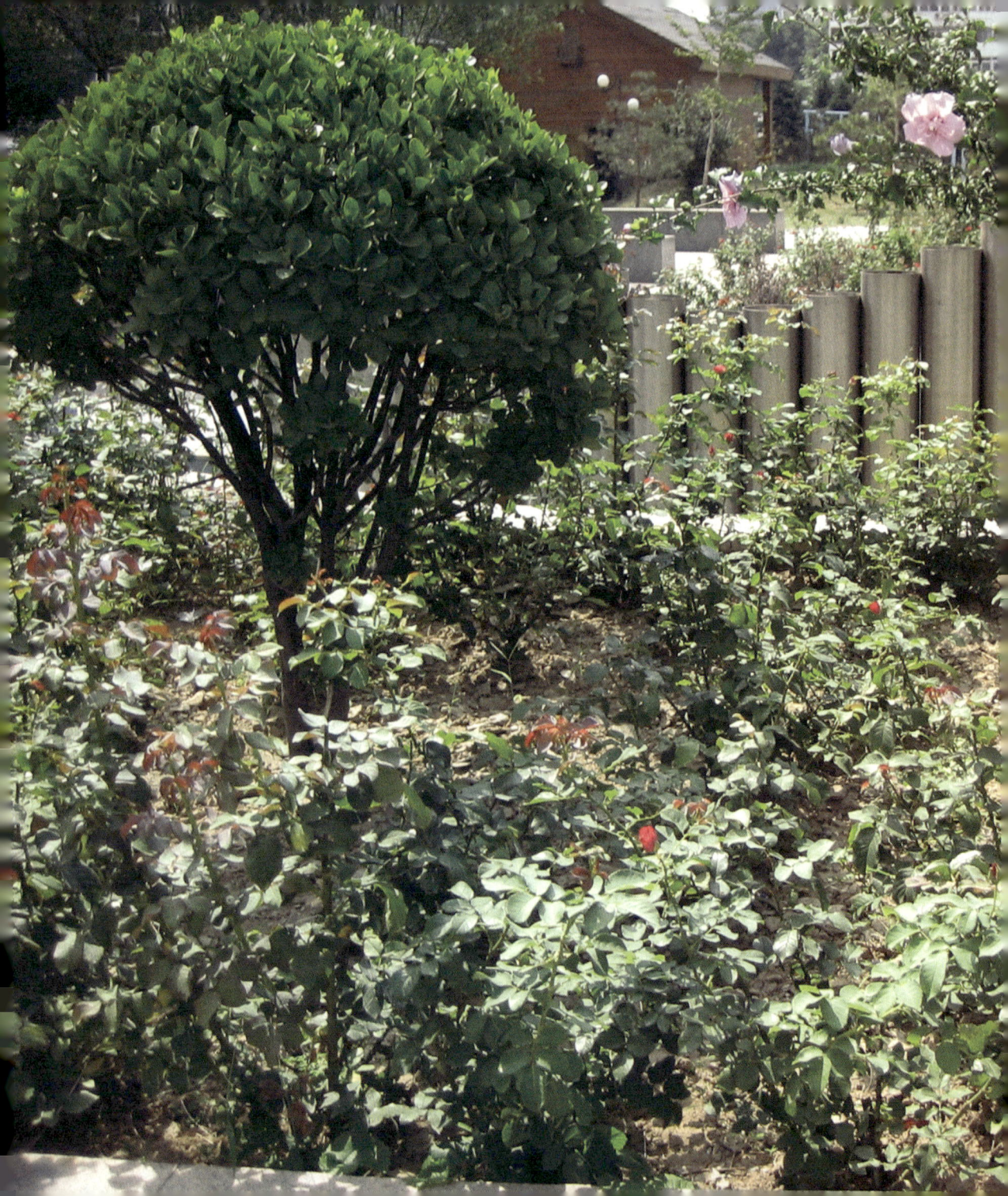

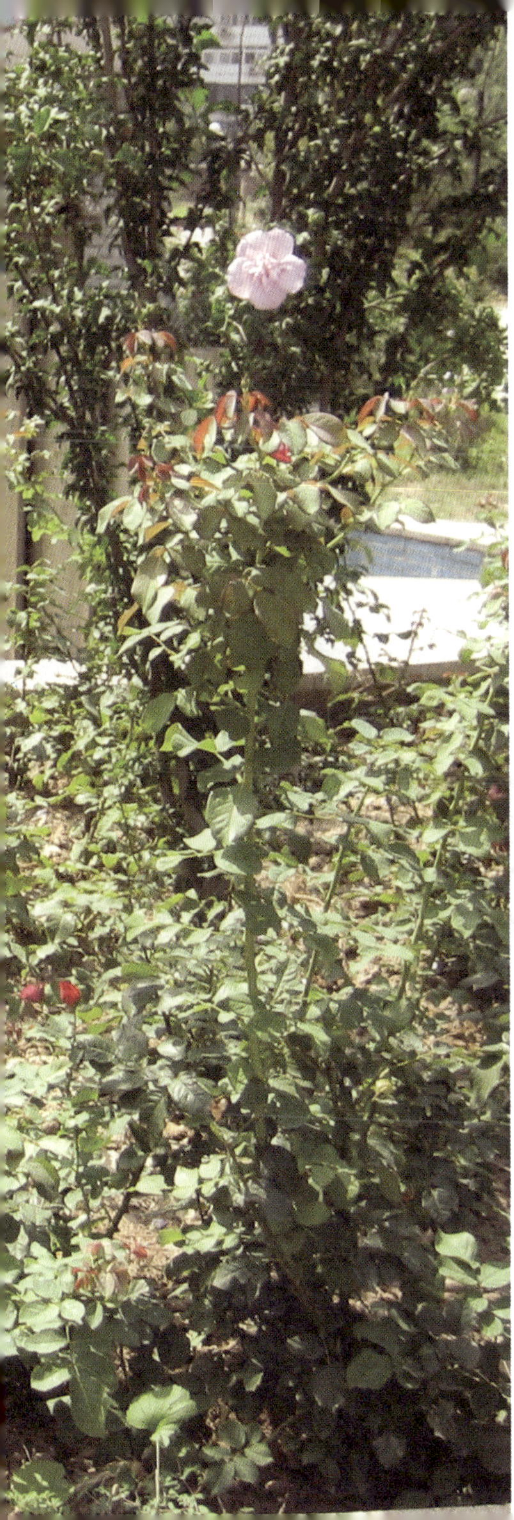

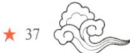

Chapter 3

How Can Diabetes Mellitus Be Prevented?

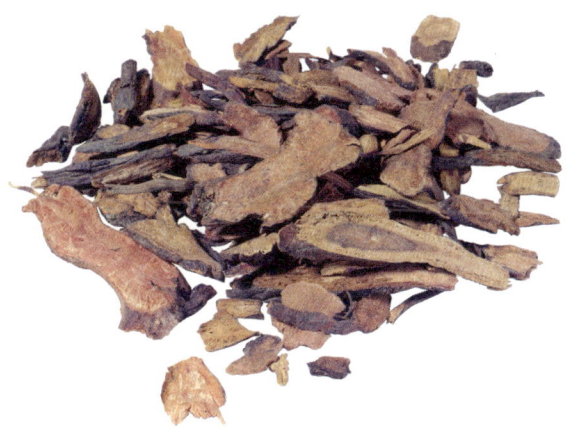

Prevention is given priority in Chinese medicine. It is commonly said that to treat disease when they have already appeared is like smithing weapons when war has already broken out, or digging a well when thirst is already severe. To effectively prevent disease, a constant balance of yin and yang is necessary. According to the *Yellow Emperor's Classic of Internal Medicine (Huáng Dì Nèi Jīng)*, staying away from pathogens, keeping good spirits, regulating your diet, and maintaining a regular lifestyle will help take care of yin and yang.

Since diabetes usually presents with yin deficiency, to prevent diabetes specifically it is necessary to protect the body's yin aspect. The following chapters will provide helpful advice to achieve end. Furthermore, attention should be paid to the established risk factors (see below).

Risk Factors for Type II Diabetes Mellitus

★ Family history of diabetes (i.e. parent of sibling with type II diabetes)
★ Obesity (BMI ≥ 25kg/m²)
★ Habitual physical inactivity
★ Race/ethnicicity (e.g. African American, Hispanic American, Native American, Asian American, Pacific Islander)
★ Previously identified IFG or IGT
★ History of GDM or delivery of baby > 4kg (>9 lb)
★ Hyptertension (blood pressure ≥ 140/90mmHg)
★ HDL cholesterol level ≥ 35mg/dl (0.09 mmol/L) and/or a triglyceride level ≥ 250mg/dl (2.82mmol/L)
★ Polycystic ovary syndrome or acanthosis nigricans
★ History of vascular disease

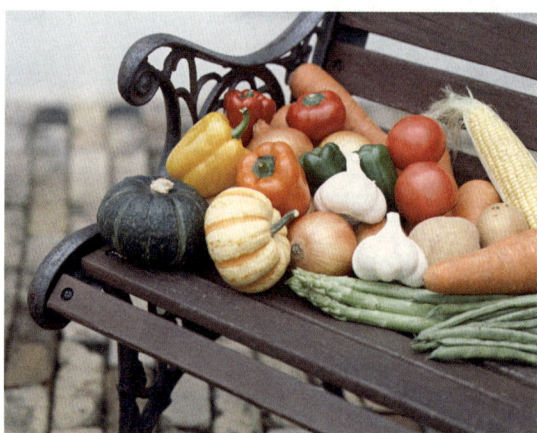

Notes: BMI, body mass index; IFG, impaired fasting glucose; IGT, impaired glucose tolerance; GDM, gestational diabetes mellitus; HDL, high-density lipoprotein.

Source: Adapted from American Diabetes Association: Standards of medical care in diabetes-2006. Diabetes Care 29 (suppl 1): S4, 2006.

So how can one maintain the balance of yin and yang in daily life?

As previously explained, all natural phenomena have yin and yang aspects, and there is a constant interaction between the human body and the natural environment. The balance is easily affected by the food you eat, your lifestyle (exercise and rest), and how you manage your emotions. Your genetic predisposition also plays a role. If you tend to be yin deficient, you can supplement yin by eating foods that nourish yin, by doing proper exercises that boost yin and preserve essence. By doing so, your body's store of yin will not become deficient and disease cannot arise.

The maintenance of psychological health is beyond the scope of this book. Chinese medicine stresses the importance of a peaceful mind for the prevention of disease. Emotional extremes most often lead to the formation of heat or fire which will eventually damage yin. Maintaining a balanced diet and getting regular exercise will go along way to maintaining a calm mind.

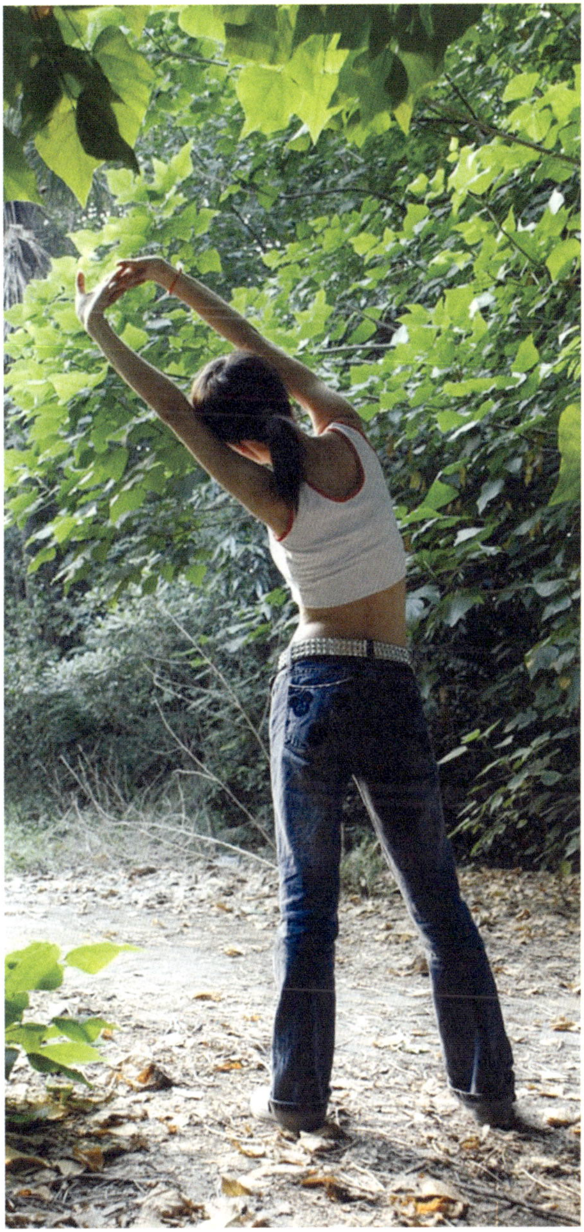

Diet

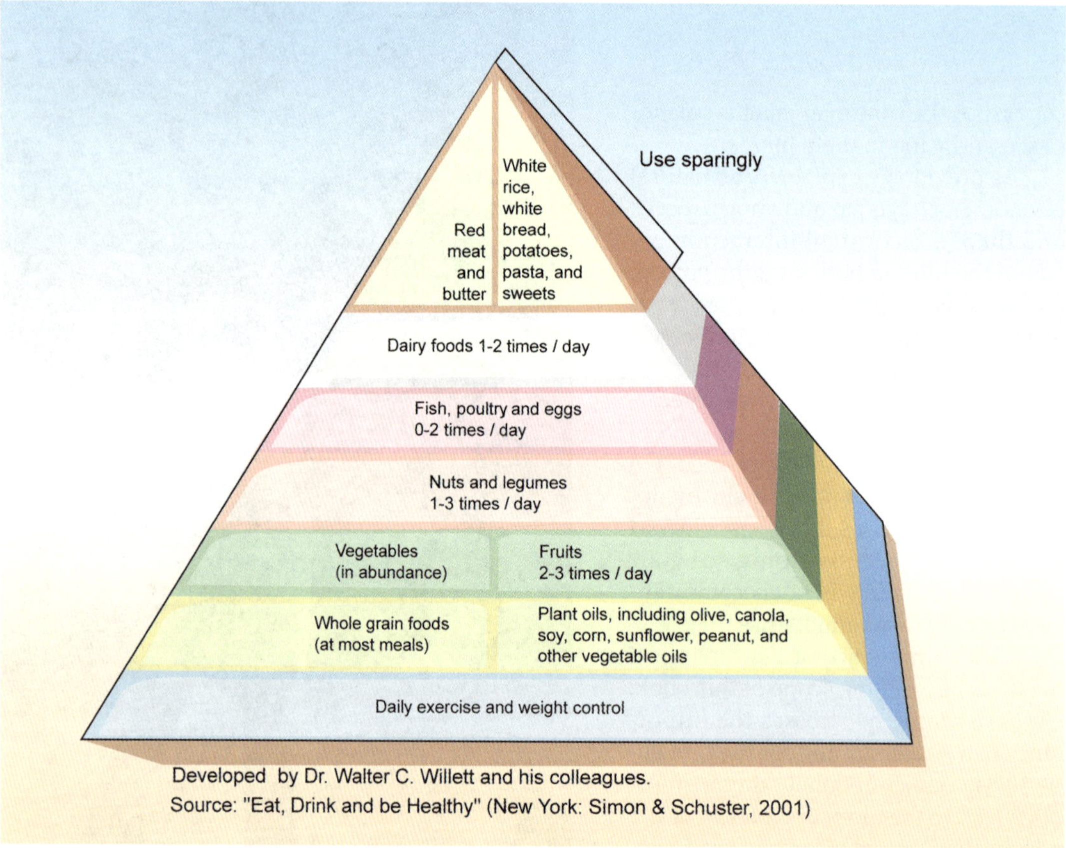

Figure 3-1 Alternative Food Pyramid

Diet is important both in the prevention and management of diabetes. The figure above is recommended by experts for ordinary people. Chinese medicine has a similar but different way to explain how to eat properly to benefit your health. To learn more, let us first learn the basics of Chinese dietary theory.

1. Essentials of Chinese Dietary Theory

Dietary therapy is essential to diabetic patients according to both biomedicine and Chinese medicine. Without proper management of your diet, insulin or any other medication won't work properly. According to Chinese medicine, food is the best medicine. The things we eat are natural substances that have their own unique qi (properties) just like Chinese medicinals. The properties of Chinese medicinals are used to correct any imbalance of qi, blood, yin, or yang. The properties of food can be used in a similar way. To some extent, it is better to use food as medicine rather than taking any kind of medication, be it Chinese medicinals or pharmaceuticals. Food is also medicinal, only that the properties of food are relatively neutral compared with medicine. Eating is also the most convenient, economic, and delicious prescription a doctor can administer.

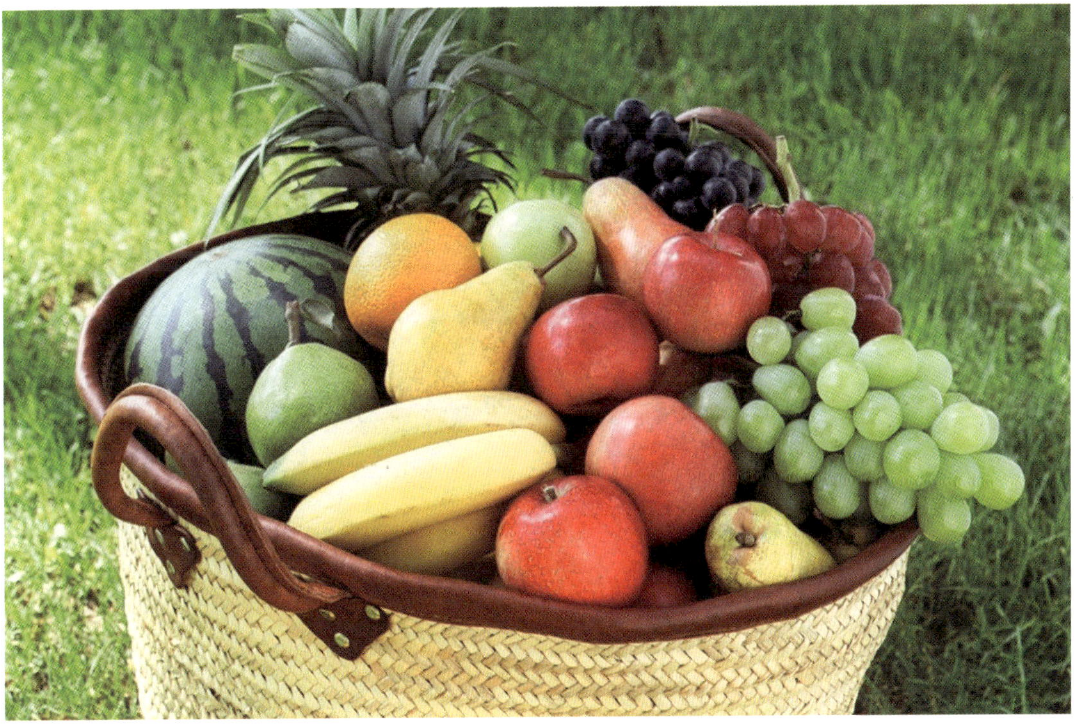

Chinese dietary theory is based on the same principles of herbal medicine. Each food has its own property and is selected based on the patient's pattern to treat disease or preserve health. Western nutritional therapy, a relatively young science, reduces food to contents that are common among all foods: carbohydrates, protein, fat, vitamins etc. It concentrates on quantity of the contents while Chinese medicine concentrates more on the qualities of each food item, dividing foods into different categories.

As an example, biomedicine would put most grains in the same category due to their high carbohydrate content. Chinese medicine, on the other hand, divides grains into different categories based on their temperature and taste. In the reverse, beef, onions, and walnuts are all considered warm in Chinese medical theory. Biomedicine on the other hand, would find little in common with these three foods. With the combination of modern nutrition and Chinese dietary theory, food therapy can be very effective.

According to Chinese medical theory, every food can be categorized as having one of the four qi (hot, warm, cool, and cold) and one or more of the five flavors (sour, bitter, sweet, spicy, and salty). This classification of food follows the same criteria used for medicinals and the application of food follows the same diagnostic principles and procedures as well. Food will act on the internal organs and influence the qi of the body, which can be used to preserve health and treat disease. The main difference that separates food from medicinal substances is that food is generally milder when compared with Chinese medicinals. That's why food can be taken daily and medicinals only once in a while when necessary.

To eat a balanced diet, in terms of Chinese medicine, is to balance the qi of the food. A diet too lopsided in one direction or the other for too long will eventually cause an imbalance of qi, blood, yin and/or yang. For those already suffering from some disease, special foods are chosen based on the patient's individual condition. Dietary prescriptions in Chinese medicine are made according to pattern identification. Biomedicine will calculate the calories, vitamins, fat content, etc. precisely. When combined, the diabetic patient can have a very well-designed dietary regimen.

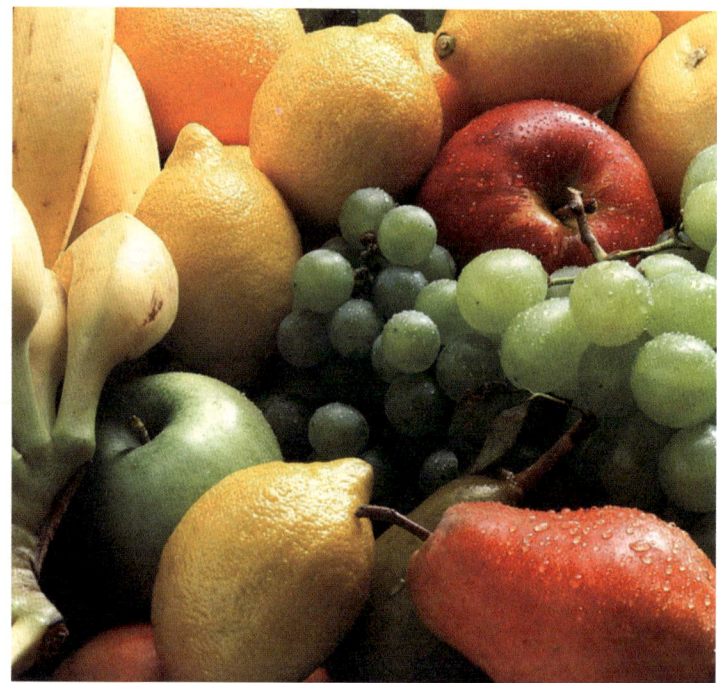

Properly chosen, food can be used as medicine. Some Chinese medicinals can be used as food and added into your diet. Indeed, many common spices (cinnamon, cardamom, ginger, garlic) are commonly used in herbal treatment. In Chinese medicine, the line between food and medicine is a blurry one. Hot foods like peppers and chilies have a warming effect on the body, while cold foods like tomatoes and bananas can cool the body. Neutral foods don't have much influence on the body, and are an important part of maintaining a healthy balance. For example, rice is neutral and thus can be consumed daily, providing nourishment while not having a drastic effect on the body's function.

The following table is an example of some common foods and their properties. A complete list of the properties of food is beyond the scope of this book. We hope that the list below will provide a good general outline, and help you make educated guesses about unlisted foods by comparing them to related items on the list.

Table 3-1 Common Foods and Their Properties

Category	Hot	Warm	Neutral	Cold	Cool
Function	Increase yang, speed up qi, warm up the body. These items tend to create heat and injure yin fluids.	Strengthen yang, warm the qi and the organs.	Build up qi and body fluids. Stabilize and harmonize the body.	Cool internal heat, calm down the spirit.	Slow down qi, clear heat, and supplement body fluids.
Beverages	Alcohol	Cocoa, Coffee, Wine		Water	Black tea, Fruit juices, Peppermint tea, Soy milk
Condiments			Honey	Salt, Soy sauce	
Dairy		Butter, Goat cheese	Cheese	Cow's milk	Yogurt
Animal products	Lamb	Beef, Eel, Chicken, Salmon	Carp, Duck, Egg, Pork, Goose	Shrimp, Crayfish	Rabbit
Fruit and vegetables		Cherry, Fennel, Leek, Peach, Onion	Carrot, Cauliflower, Grape, Plum, Potato	Asparagus, Banana, Orange, Rhubarb, Seaweed, Tomato, Watermelon	Celery, Cucumber, Soy bean, Sprouts, Spinach, Zucchini
Grains and legumes			Corn, Lentil, Millet, Peas, Rice, Spelt		Barley, Tofu, Wheat
Herbs and spices	Cinnamon, Chili, Curry, Garlic, Ginger, Paprika, Pepper	Anise, Basil, Rosemary		Dandelion, Yellow gentian	Tarragon
Nuts		Walnut	Hazelnut		

(The table is adapted from P23, Joweh Kastner. Chinese Nutrition Therapy. Thieme Stuttgart, New York, 2004)

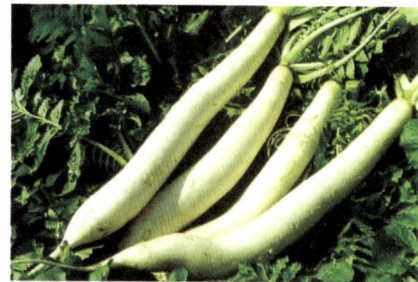
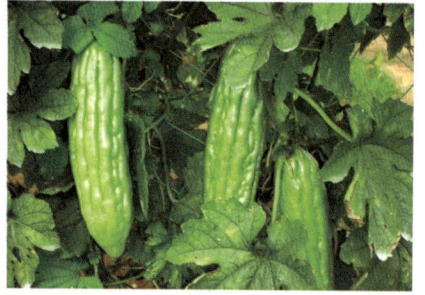
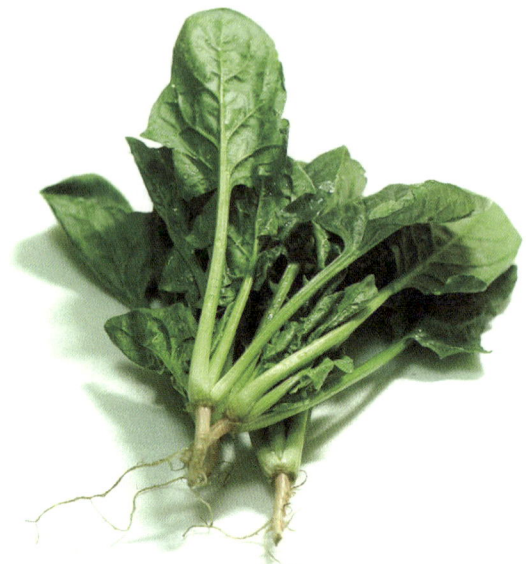

The flavors of foods are associated with the internal organs, and influence them just like medicinals do. The essence of Chinese dietary therapy is to make proper food choices and add medicinals into the diet that will help to restore your body's harmony. Since the typical root pattern of diabetes is internal heat due to yin deficiency, patients are recommended to eat food that is cool or cold to clear the heat, supplement yin, and produce fluids. For example: spinach, turnip, bitter melon, white gourd, millet, common (white) yam, kiwi, tomato, water chestnut, sea cucumber, duck, goose, rabbit, and milk. Hot and spicy foods should be avoided. Some of these foods are: alcohol, ginger, garlic, hot spices, etc.

2. Specifics and Recipes for Diabetes

Special items for Diabetes

The following items are cool or cold in nature. They are highly recommended by Chinese medicine practitioners for patients with diabetes. Many of these foods are not common to the western diet. But because they are so helpful in preventing and treating disease, patients are strongly advised to find these wonderful foods and integrate them into their diets. Many of them can be found in Asian supermarkets or natural food stores. Some of them are available in concentrated form as pills or powders. In order to help you find them, we have tried to include various common names, as well as the Chinese characters.

1) Bitter Melon – 苦瓜 *(kǔ guā)*

Despite its bitter taste, this vegetable is extremely beneficial to diabetes patients. If you find you can't get used to the taste, bitter melon is available in pill form from many health food stores. As with any medicine, make sure you buy from a reputable brand.

As its name suggests, the taste is quite bitter and can be difficult to get used to. Those who like it enjoy it stir fried with onion, egg, and chicken, or cooked in a soup with noodles and other vegetables.

Bitter melon is bitter in taste, cold in nature, and can clear heat, remove toxins, calm the spirit, and quench thirst.

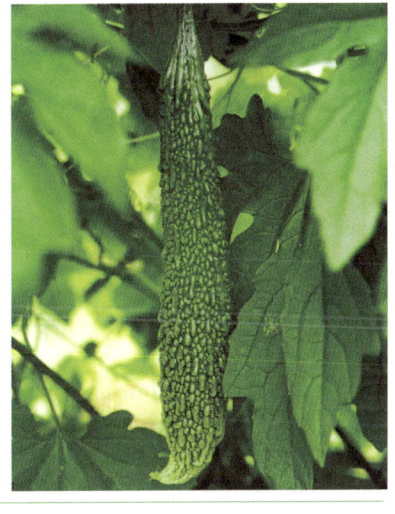

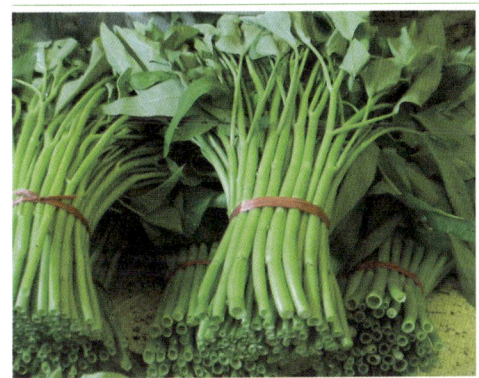

2) Water Spinach – 空心菜 *(kōng xīn cài)*

Sometimes known by its Cantonese name "Ong Choy" in western countries, this resilient plant grows in water and needs no pesticides. It is rich in cellulose, vitamins, and minerals. Eating it regularly can lower blood sugar levels. Patients with weak or cold constitutions are advised not to eat it too often. Water spinach can be prepared like any other green leafy vegetable, steaming, stir-frying, adding to soups, etc.

3) Gold Theragran – 绞股蓝 *(jiǎo gǔ lán)*

Another name for gold theragran is southern ginseng. It contains proteins, vitamins, flavonoids, and panaxsaponin (the major active ingredient of ginseng). It has the effect of boosting immunity, relieving fatigue, and lowering blood sugar. There is no report of any side-effects due to long term consumption. Gold theragran is usually taken alone as a simple tea or consumed as a dietary supplement in pill form, and is popular in China, Japan, and Korea.

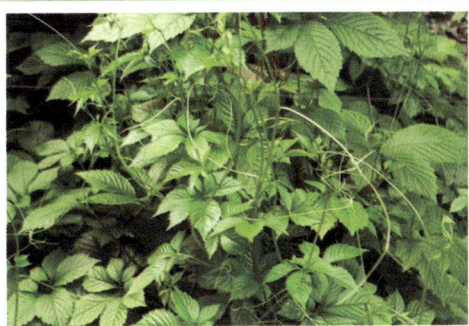

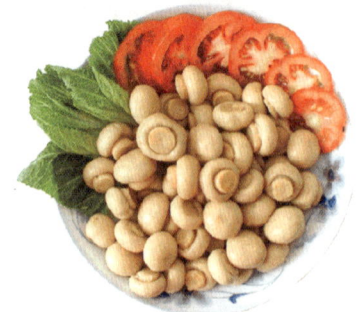

4) Mushrooms – 蘑菇 (mó gū)

These common and delicious fungi are rich in proteins, polysaccharides, and trace elements. They can calm the mind, lower blood pressure, boost immunity, relieve fatigue, and decrease blood sugar. They are especially good for diabetic patients who are very thin. Recently Hericium Erinaceus, commonly called Lion's Mane Mushroom, has been found to have substances called glucosans, which are proven to be effective in lowering blood sugar levels.

5) Amorphophallus Konjac – 魔芋 (mó yú)

Amorphophallus konjac, more commonly known by its Japanese name "Konyaku" and usually sold as a type of Japanese food, is rich in amino acids, minerals and alkaloids. The effective ingredient it contains called mannan can lower blood sugar levels.

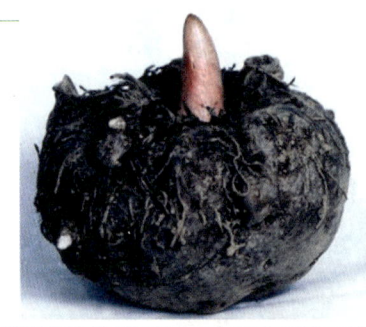

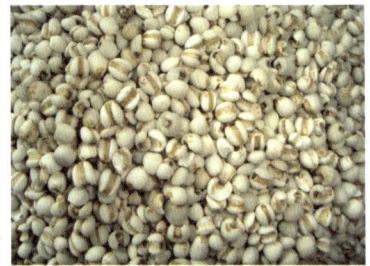

6) Chinese White and Black Fungus – 木耳 (mù ěr)

These common ingredients in Chinese cooking are rich in protein and fiber. The acidic polysaccharose these fungi contain can improve pancreas cell function and lower blood sugar levels.

7) Coix Seed – 薏仁 (yì rén)

Also known by the poetic name "Job's Tears Seeds", these small grains can be used similar to rice or barley. The amount of carbohydrates in coix is lower than in rice, while the protein and vitamin content are three times that of rice. The major components, coixol and terpenoids, are anti-cancer, diuretic, and can lower blood sugar. It is especially indicated for diabetic patients with hypertension who suffer form excessive urination and are overweight.

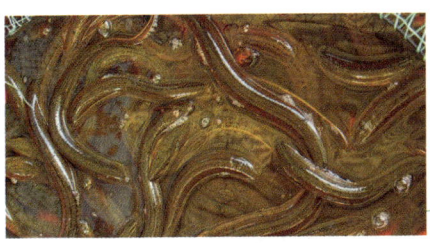

8) Eel – 鳝鱼 *(shàn yú)*

Eels are warm in nature and sweet in flavor. Eating them can strengthen digestion and move stagnant qi and blood. They help the kidneys and lungs and can also lower blood sugar levels.

9) Pig Pancreas – 猪胰 *(zhū yí)*

This item probably sounds very unusual to most non-Chinese patients, but we have listed it here because it is the classic home remedy for diabetes. It is neutral and sweet and can strengthen the digestion and generate fluids. It can be cooked like any meat product, but in China it is available as a supplement in pill form. In fact, in the past the insulin diabetes patients injected was often from pigs. And recently there has been experiments attempting to implant cells from very young pig pancreas into rats to treat diabetes, the experiments have had some success.

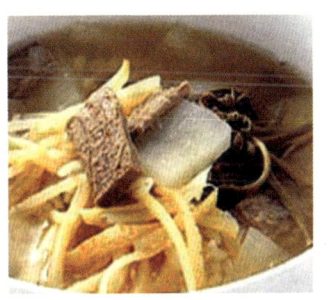

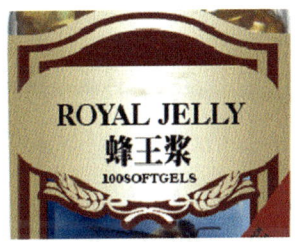

10) Royal Jelly – 蜂王浆 *(fēng wáng jiāng)*

This product is commonly found in natural food stores and Asian supermarkets around the world. It is cool, sour, and slightly sweet. The unsaturated fatty acids and polypeptides it contains can boost immunity, regulate the endocrine system, and lower blood sugar.

*Everyday Eating

Below are some suggestions on medicinal ingredients that can be used in simple recipes plus common foods that are good for diabetics. They are also indicated for those who are concerned about being diabetic. The information is categorized by the most commonly seen patterns that were described in previous chapters. Most of the medicinals cited are sweet flavored or fairly bland so they won't impart a very strong taste to the dishes. Most of them are best used in soups and stews, though more specific cooking information is listed in the recipes. The patterns listed below are simple ones and a patient may have two or more of the patterns mentioned below. If that is the case, please choose freely from either list. We hope that with the advice of your practitioner, you can learn which recipes and ingredients are right for you and incorporate them into your daily routine. You should be able to buy the medicinals in small amounts to be used in cooking from your practitioner or in an Asian supermarket.

*Notice: Please consult your practitioner for food choices that fit your pattern.

Recipes for Different Patterns
1) Yin deficiency

<Signs and Symptoms> a high thirst, dry mouth, dry stool, dark colored urine, a red tongue with little coating, and a fine rapid pulse

Table 3-2 Medicinals to use in cooking for yin deficiency

Medicinals	Pinyin	Latin Name
Rehmannia Root	shēng dì huáng	Radix Rehmanniae Recens
Wolfberry Fruit/Gou Ji Berries	gǒu qǐ zǐ	Fructus Lycii
Kudzu Root	gě gēn	Radix Puerariae Lobatae
Common Yam Rhizome/Yam	shān yào	Rhizoma Dioscoreae

<Food Items> Yam, Bitter Melon, Black Sesame, Rabbit, Honey, Rice Porridge

<Recommended Recipes>

Fragrant Solomonseal Rhizome cooked with lotus root
Use 30-60g of Fragrant Solomonseal Rhizome. Place it in a pot with boiling water. Cook it for 5 minutes and drain the water. Cook lotus roots slices with boiling water for a few seconds and drain this water also. Add vegetable oil into a skillet and put the Fragrant Solomonseal Rhizome and lotus root slice into it. Cook for a while and add salt, ginger juice and pepper powder when it is ready.

Pig pancreas (or simply pork) cooked with common yam
Use 60g of yam and one pig pancreas (or 200g pork). Add salt and other desired seasonings, and stew in a small amount of water until both ingredients are well cooked and most of the water is boiled off.

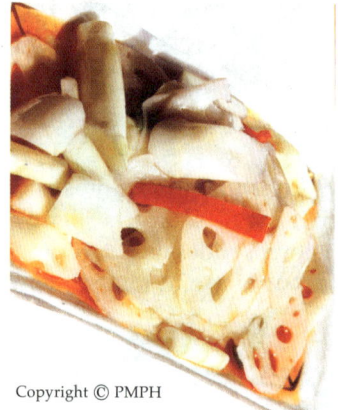

Copyright © PMPH

Fragrant Solomonseal Rhizome Cooked with Lotus Root

Chinese black fungus cooked with tofu skin (yuba)
Use 100g Chinese black fungus and 100g yuba. Cut into small pieces. Add cooking wine and some lean pork slices and marinate for a while. Add some oil into a pot and start stir frying green onion and yuba. Add the Chinese black fungus and pork and cook it for a while. Add some salt, chicken broth, and other desired seasonings. Eat when all ingredients are cooked through.

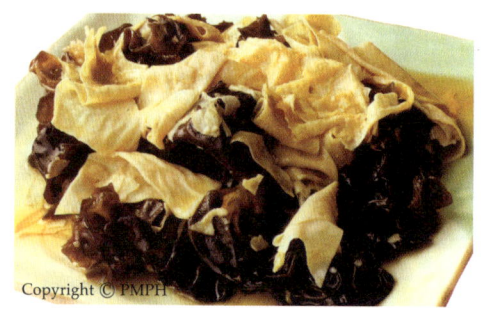

Copyright © PMPH

Chinese Black Fungus Cooked with Tofu Skin (YuBa)

2) Qi deficiency

<Signs and Symptoms> fatigue, lassitude, abdominal bloating, loose stool, a pale tongue with a white coating, and a fine weak pulse

Table 3-3 Medicinals to use in cooking for qi deficiency

Medicinals	Pinyin	Latin Name
Ginseng	rén shēn	Radix et Rhizoma Ginseng
Milkvetch Root/Astragalus	huáng qí	Radix Astragali
Common Yam Rhizome	shān yào	Rhizoma Dioscoreae
Poria	fú líng	Poria
Lotus Seed	lián zǐ	Semen Nelumbinis
Gordon Euryale Seed	qiàn shí	Semen Euryales

<Food Items> Pumpkin, Bee Pollen, Tofu, Common Yam, Soy Beans

<Recommended Recipes>

Rice porridge with common yam and lotus seed

Boil a suitable amount of rice, yam, and lotus seeds until all are very soft. The final consistency should be of a thick soup.

Rice porridge with astragalus and common yam

Boil a suitable amount of rice, yam, and astragalus until all are very soft. The final consistency should be of a thick soup. Normally the astragalus isn't eaten, but its properties will be transferred to the porridge during cooking.

Duck cooked with gordon euryale seeds

Stuff an aged duck with 120 grams of gordon euryale seeds. Place in a pot and cover with water, and add green onion, ginger, and salt. You may add vegetables if you like. Cook until duck is done and the seeds are soft.

Beef cooked with winter bamboo shoots

Use 75g winter bamboo shoot and 100g beef (250g cactus can be used if available). Shred the above ingredients separately. Mix shredded beef with cooking wine and mix well. Place oil into pot and heat it. Add the beef first and cook until the color changes. Add winter bamboo shoot (and cactus). Finally add salt, pepper, and other desired seasoning.

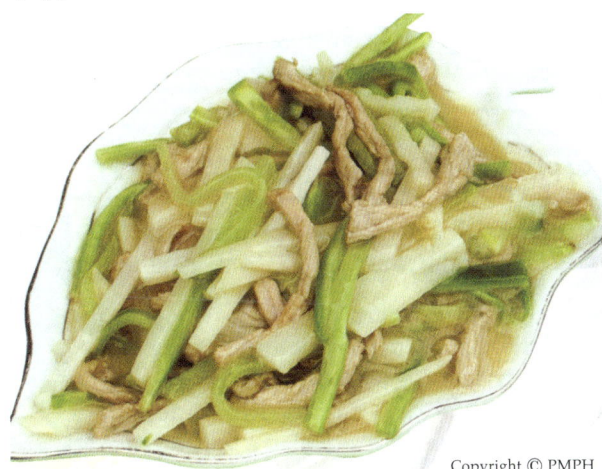

Beef Cooked with Winter Bamboo Shoots

3) Deficiency of qi and yin

<Signs and Symptoms> a combination of the signs and symptoms listed under qi deficiency and yin deficiency above

Table 3-4 Medicinals to use in cooking for deficiency of qi and yin

Medicinals	Pinyin	Latin Name
Ginseng	rén shēn	Radix et Rhizoma Ginseng
Milkvetch Root/Astragalus	huáng qí	Radix Astragali
American Ginseng	xī yáng shēn	Radix Panacis Quinquefolii
Wolfberry Fruit/Gou Qi Berries	gǒu qǐ zǐ	Lycii Fructus
Rehmannia Root	shēng dì huáng	Radix Rehmanniae Recens
Solomonseal Rhizome	huáng jīng	Rhizoma Polygonat

<Food Items> Spinach, Raddish, White Gourd, Corn, Yam, Kiwi Fruit, Water Chestnut, Chicken, Duck, Milk

<Recommended Recipes>

Ginseng and wolfberry (gou qi) fruit tea
Boil 3-6 grams (a small handful) each of ginseng and wolfberry in two cups of water for about 30 minutes.

Pig pancreas cooked with ginseng
Boil 5-10g of ginseng and about 150g of pig pancreas together. Add salt when the meat is cooked. Eat the pancreas and drink the soup.

Pork cooked with cucumber
Slice 350g cucumber and 100g pork separately. Cut 50g Chinese black fungus into pieces. Mix pork with cooking wine and marinate for a while. Add oil to a pot and heat it. Cook the meat until the color changes. Add Chinese black fungus. Remove from heat and add cucumber, salt, and other desired seasonings.

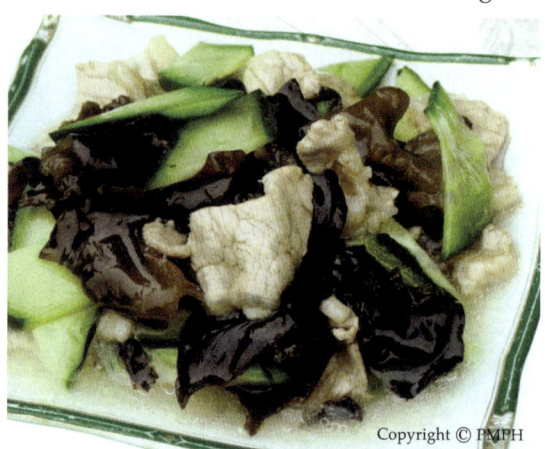

Pork Cooked with Cucumber

4) Deficiency of yin and yang

<Signs and Symptoms> fatigue, weakness, soreness in the low back and knees, feverish sensation on the palms and soles, a cold sensation on the backs of the palms and soles, a pale tongue, and a deep fine pulse

Table 3-5 Medicinals to Use in Cooking for Deficiency of Yin and Yang

Medicinals	Pinyin	Latin Name
Cinnamon	ròu guì	Cortex Cinnamomi
Sliced Cornu Cervi	lù jiǎo	Cornu Cervi
Wolfberry Fruit/Gou Qi Berries	gǒu qǐ zǐ	Lycii Fructus
Ginseng	rén shēn	Radix et Rhizoma Ginseng
Herba Epimedii	yín yáng huò	Herba Epimedii
Milkvetch Root	huáng qí	Radix Astragali
GreenOnion/Rehmannia Root	dì huáng	Radix Rehmanniae

<Recommended Recipes>

Ginseng tea with wolfberry (gou qi) fruit and herba epimedii

Boil 3-6 grams (a small handful) each of ginseng, wolfberry, and epimedii leaves in two cups of water for about 30 minutes.

Pancreas cooked with onions

Put the pancreas into boiling water for a few seconds then take it out and slice it. Add cooking wine, ginger juice, and salt and marinate for 15 minutes. Slice about 150g of onions and stir-fry in oil. Add the pancreas slices and other flavors and cook until the meat is done.

Walnut and black bean porridge

Wash 50g black bean and 100g millet. Cook it with 30g walnuts and water until the consistency is thick and all the ingredients are cooked well.

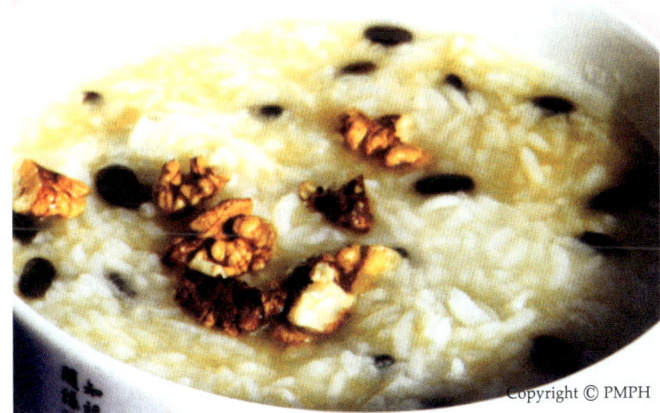

Walnut and Black Bean Porridge

5) Liver fire flaring

<Signs and Symptoms> dizziness, vertigo, headache, and red or sore eyes

Table 3-6 Medicinals to Use in Cooking for Liver Fire Flaring

Medicinals	*Pinyin*	Latin Name
Mulberry Leaf	*sāng yè*	Folium Mori
Chrysanthemum Flower	*jú huā*	Floschrysanthemi
Cassia Seed	*jué míng zǐ*	Semen Cassiae
Broadleaf Holly Leaf	*kǔ dīng*	Herbacorydalis Bungeanae

<Recommended Recipes>

Tea

These medicinals are generally made as a tea. Simply steep a small amount of any one in a teapot and enjoy.

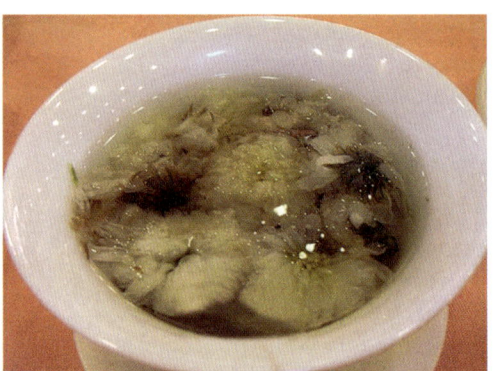

Chrysanthemum Flower Tea

6) Accumulated heat in the stomach and intestines

<Signs and Symptoms> thirst, constipation

<Medicinals to use in cooking>
Senna Leaf

<Food Items> Bitter Melon, Amorphophallus Konjac (konyaku), Radish, Pumpkin, Lotus Root, Pear, Water Chestnut, Tomato, Bottle Gourd, Buckwheat.

< Recommended Recipes>
Bitter melon cooked with pork
Slice some lean pork. Add cooking wine, soy sauce, a little sugar, and starch and marinate for a while. Put sliced bitter melon (seeds removed) into boiling water for 1 minute. Take out and place in a bowl of cool water. Fry the pork slices with oil until almost cooked. Put the pork aside. Add more oil to the pan, when hot add garlic, ginger and black bean sauce. Then add the bitter melon and pork. Stir-fry it for a few more minutes until done.

Senna leaf tea
A very small amount of senna leaves boiled for 5 minutes in a cup of water. Senna tea bags can often be bought in natural food stores.

Tofu and edible rape
Wash 50g dried tofu and 200g rape. Put 5g oil into the pot and heat it. Add rape and shredded dried tofu. Add salt, green onion, and ground pepper. Any green vegetable may be used in this recipe.

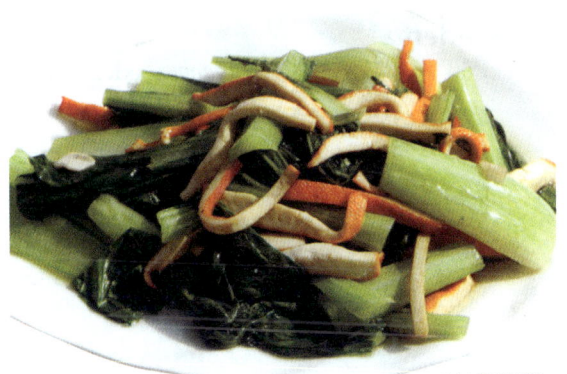

Tofu and Edible Rape

7) Blood stasis
<Signs and Symptoms> chest pain or other severe localized pain, a dark tongue, and purple lips

Table 3-7 Medicinals to Use in Cooking for Blood Stasis

Medicinals	*Pinyin*	Latin Name
Hawthorn Fruit	shān zhā	Fructus Crataegi
Kudzu Root	gě gēn	Radix Puerariae Lobatae
Peach Seed	táo rén	Semen Persicae
Seaweed	hǎi zǎo	Sargassum

<Food Items> Eggplant, Lotus Root, Rose Tea, Purple Stemmed Choi Sum

< Recommended Recipes>
Hawthorn fruit and wolfberry (gou qi) tea
Boil 3-6 grams (a small handful) each of hawthorn and wolfberry in two cups of water for about 30 minutes.

White chicken cooked with hawthorn fruit and wolfberry (gou qi)
Put 30g hawthorn fruit, 10g gouji and 150g white chicken meat together. Add water and cook until the chicken is done. Add salt and other desired spices.

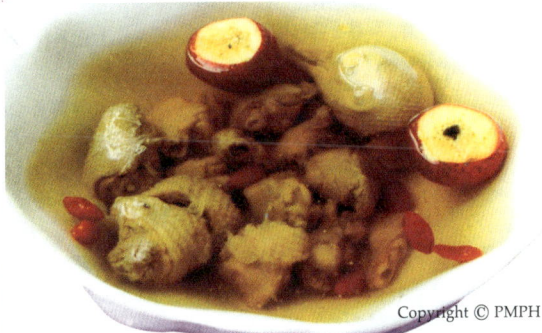

Hawthorn Fruit and Wolfberry (Gou Qi) Tea

8) Edema

<Signs and Symptoms> edema, difficulty or scanty urination

Table 3-8 Medicinals to use in cooking for edema

Medicinals	Pinyin	Latin Name
Chinese wax gourd peel	dōng guā pí	Exocarpium Benincasae
Dried tangerine peel	chén pí	Pericarpium Citri Reticulatae
White mulberry root-bark	sāng bái pí	Mori Cortex
Bottle-gourd peel	hú lú pí	Lagenaria Siceraria

<Food Items> Corn, Adzuki Bean, Ginger Peel, Carp

<Recommended Recipes>

Carp soup

Wash and clean the carp. Fry the carp in oil until golden brown. Add water and flavor with cooking wine, salt, sugar, green onion, ginger, and other spices depending on your taste. Cook until the carp is ready. Take out the ginger and green onion. Add pepper and enjoy.

Celery cooked with mushroom

Use 200g celery (cut into pieces), 50g mushroom (shredded), and 20g peppers (shredded). Place 5g vegetable oil into the pot and add green onion when the oil is hot. Add celery, cayenne pepper and mushroom. Cook them together until tender. Add salt and other desired spices.

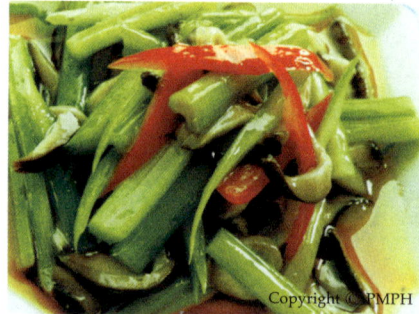
Celery cooked with mushroom

Celery cooked with tomato and eggplant

Use 100g celery pieces, 100g shredded eggplant and 100g tomato pieces. Put celery and eggplant into boiling water for a few minutes and take them out. Add tomato pieces. Add salt, olive oil, green onion, and a little sugar. Mix them up and it is ready to eat.

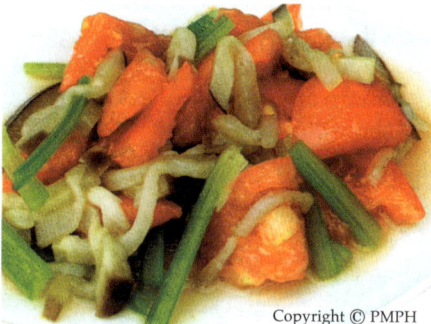
Celery Cooked with Tomato and Eggplant

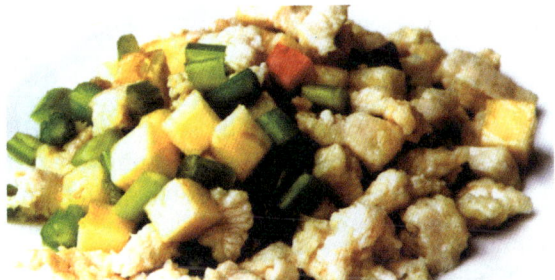

Chicken cooked with pineapple and pepper
Cut 20g pineapple into cubes and keep the juice. Cut 30g chicken breast into cubes. Mix the chicken with 50ml pineapple juice and some salt. Marinate for a while. Add olive oil into a pot and heat it. Add 30g green onion and then the chicken. Add red and green peppers. Add the pineapple. Cook for a few seconds. Turn off the fire. Add salt and other desired spices. Then it's ready!

Chicken Cooked with Pineapple and Pepper

Food recommended for diabetic patients for everyday eating

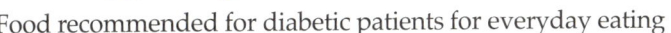

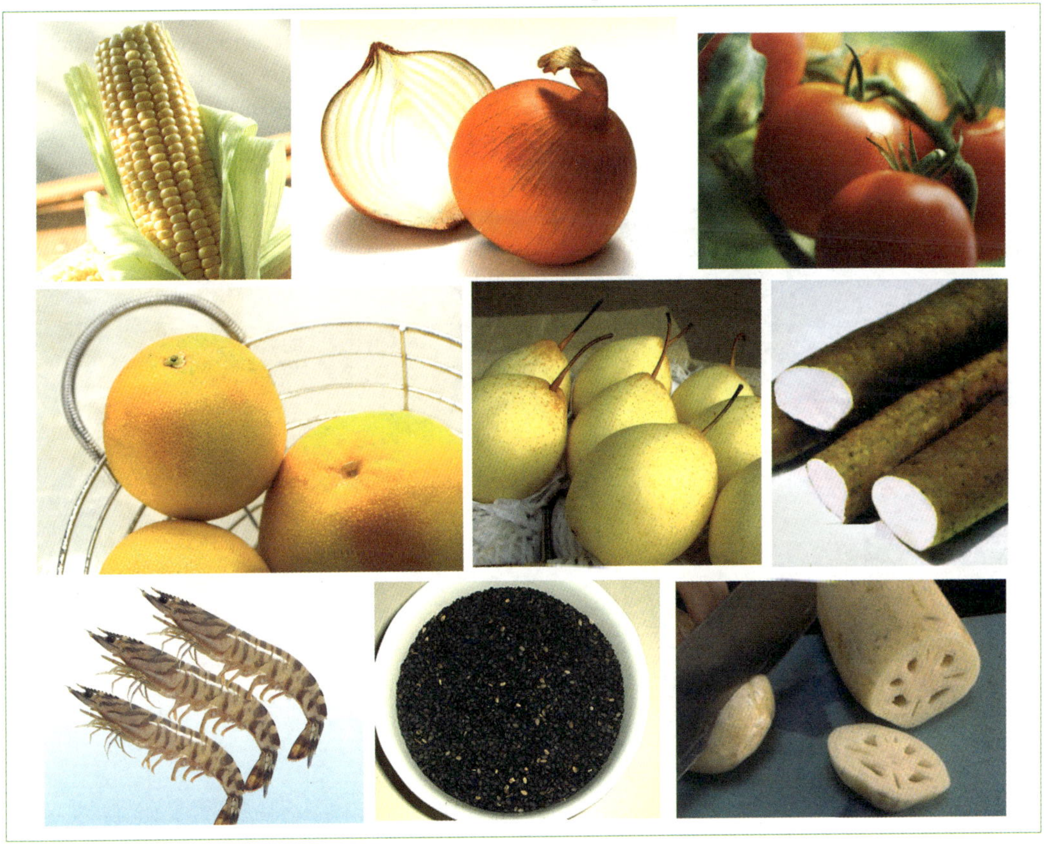

A Legend

Once upon a time in China, there was a scholar on his way to the capital to take part in the national civil service examination. To get there from his village he had to walk for several months. Along the way he didn't eat well and tired himself out from walking all day. Eventually he got sick and had to stop and see a doctor along the way. The doctor saw right away that the scholar had "*xiao ke*" (which most likely meant he had diabetes). The doctor knew the scholar wanted to do well on his exam and didn't want to worry him, so the doctor didn't tell him how serious his disease was. Instead, the wise old doctor recommended the scholar take another route to the capital, along which grew pear trees for hundreds of miles. Whenever the scholar felt thirsty, the doctor told him to eat the pears. The scholar took the doctor's advice and ate pears all the way to the capital. When he arrived his disease was gone. Healthy and calm, and he passed the examination.

Pears are considered cold and sweet in Chinese dietary theory. They can clear heat, produce fluids, supplement yin, and moisturize the lungs. Pears contain carbohydrates, vitamins and organic acid. The main carbohydrate in pears is fructose, which has little influence on blood sugar levels after meals. So it is perfect for diabetic patients. One should choose a pear that is juicy but not too sweet. There is an old recipe for *xiao ke* (diabetes) in Chinese medicine that uses the juice from five different plants, the pear is one of the ingredients.

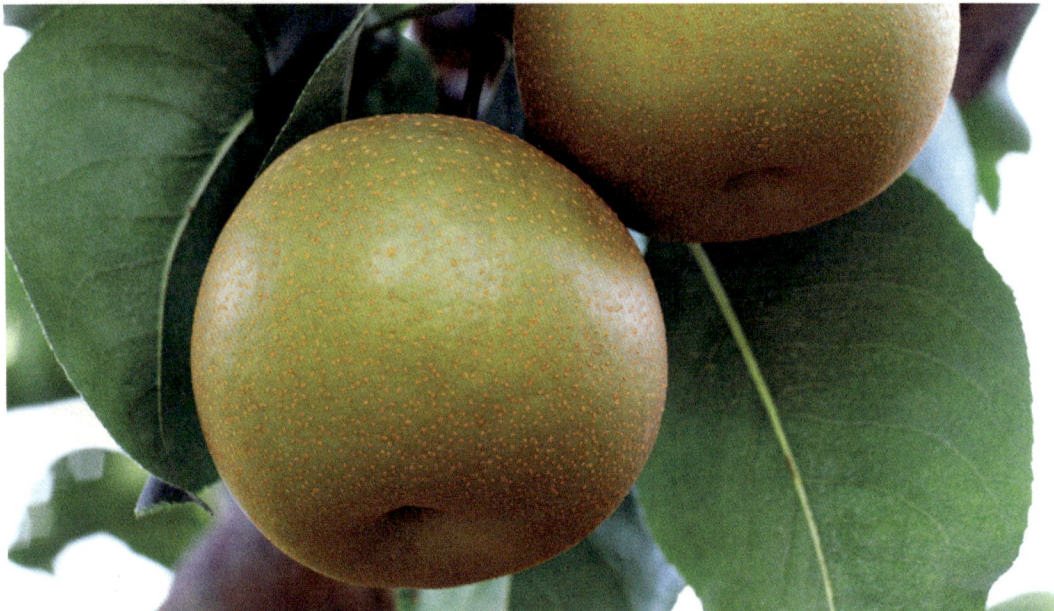

Exercise (Tai Ji Quan, Qi Gong)

1. What Kinds of Exercises Are Helpful and What Should Be Avoided?

Exercise is essential to one's health. This is no exception to Chinese medicine or biomedicine. To reduce your risks of chronic disease, you had better put yourself on a schedule of regular exercise. Physical activity is one of the most beneficial therapies for patients with diabetes. Together with medication and dietary therapy it is an essential part of the successful management of diabetes. In this part, you will read how Chinese medicine thinks of exercise in the management of diabetes and its unique exercises of tai ji quan and qi gong.

From ancient times, Chinese medicine has advocated exercise as a way to treat diabetes. A book *General Treatise on Causes and Manifestations of All Diseases* (*Zhū Bìng Yuán Hóu Lùn*) written by Chao Yuan-fang in the Sui Dynasty (581-681 A.D.) says that diabetic patients should walk 120 to 1000 steps before meals. While another book, the *Medical Secrets of a Frontier Official* (*Wài Tái Mì Yào*) written by Wang Tao in the Tang Dynasty (618-907 A.D.) suggests that diabetic patients "should walk after meals" and "exercise moderately without straining or going to extremes".

Although there is inconsistent scientific evidence that routine exercise will improve glucose control in type I diabetes, there is evidence that shows improved glucose control in individuals with type II diabetes. Nevertheless, patients with both type I and type II will benefit from regular exercise.

If you have type II diabetes, are overweight, and have blood sugar levels ranging from 11.1-16.7mmol/L(200 - 300mg/dl), or if your type I diabetes is under control, then it is highly recommended that you engage in regular exercises like walking, swimming, jogging, cycling etc. Of course, after reading this chapter you may want to try tai ji quan or qi gong, which are both healthy and healing.

However, if your diabetes is serious with severe complications, or if you have symptoms of no appetite, vomiting, or diarrhea, we suggest you avoid excessive exercise.

When you exercise, make sure to bring some biscuits or sugar with you in case hypoglycemia is induced by the activity.

As to what kinds of exercises are appropriate, the first principle is to choose one that won't strain you excessively or make you overly tired. Another equally important principle is to choose one you like!

Walking is a good recommendation. Other good choices are hiking, cycling, swimming, or tai ji quan. You are not supposed to exercise to exhaustion. The best time to exercise is one hour after a meal. Try your best not to exercise alone and keep an eye on your blood pressure, heart beat, and blood sugar. Exercise regularly and constantly for the most benefit.

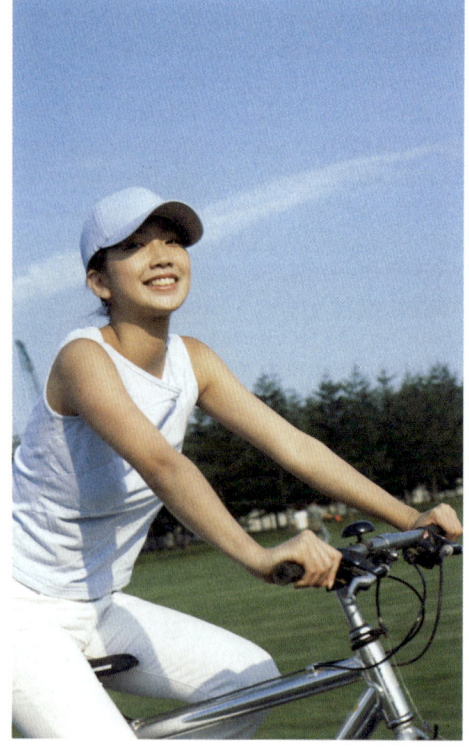

2. Tai Ji Quan and Qi Gong

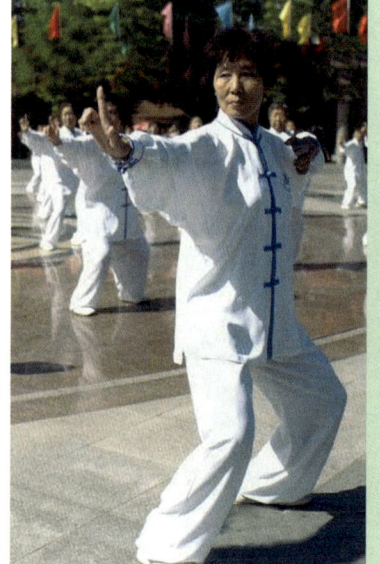

Tai ji quan and qi gong are great exercises to improve your health and body's function to prevent diseases. It is especially helpful for chronic diseases like diabetes.

Tai ji quan

Tai ji quan (quan literally means fist), a unique body-mind exercise, is a martial art based on Daoist philosophy and yin-yang theory. It is a special kind of kung fu practiced to maintain health and for self-defense. It is suitable for both young and old, and makes a great aerobic exercise that doesn't demand a lot of bodily energy or strength to learn. The more you practice, the better you will understand your own body. It helps to coordinate and clear your body and mind. You will feel peace and grace physically, psychologically, and emotionally after practicing tai ji quan. Modern research has shown it to boost immunity, and it can help diabetic patients to reduce blood sugar levels and improve their overall sense of well-being.

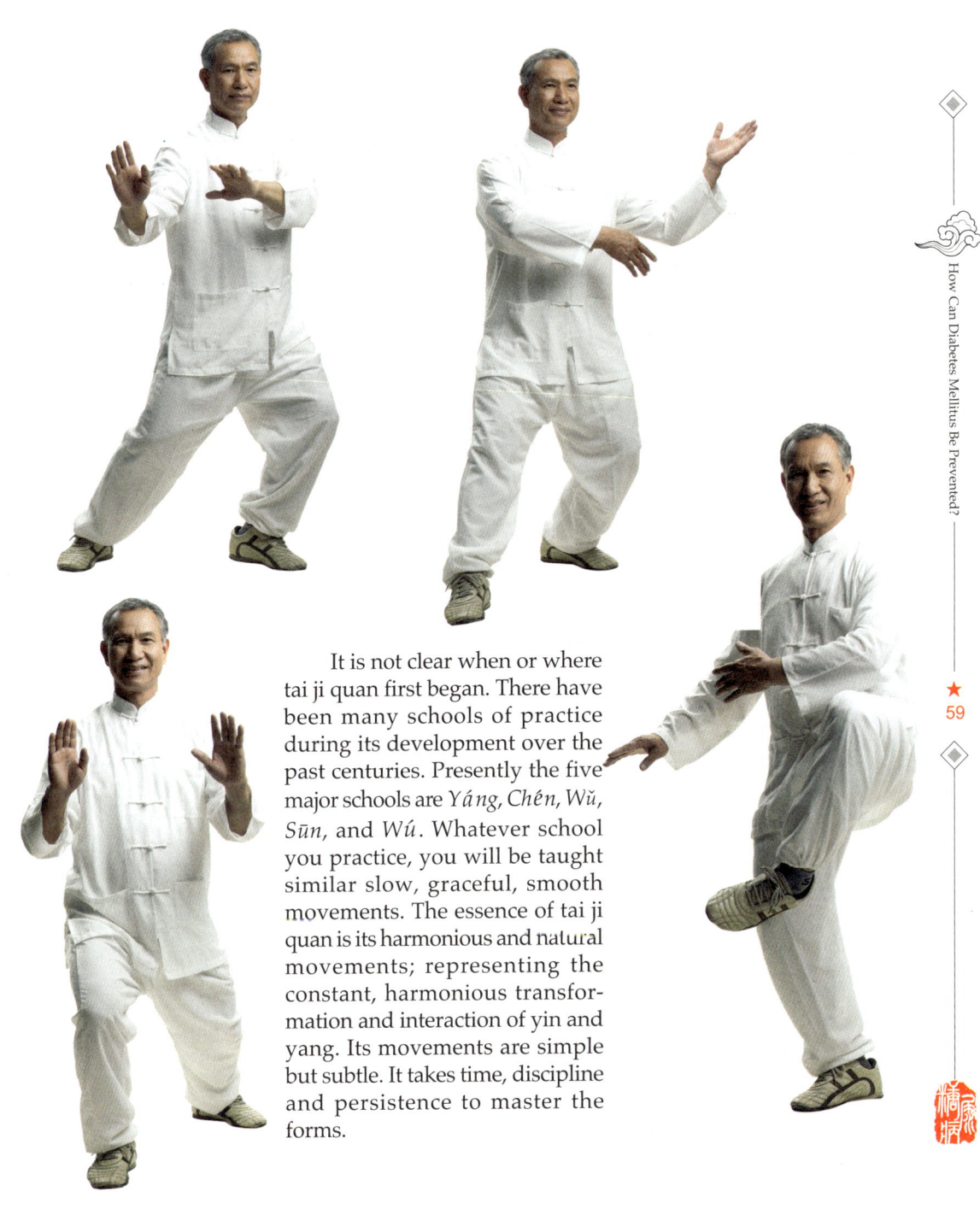

It is not clear when or where tai ji quan first began. There have been many schools of practice during its development over the past centuries. Presently the five major schools are *Yáng*, *Chén*, *Wǔ*, *Sūn*, and *Wú*. Whatever school you practice, you will be taught similar slow, graceful, smooth movements. The essence of tai ji quan is its harmonious and natural movements; representing the constant, harmonious transformation and interaction of yin and yang. Its movements are simple but subtle. It takes time, discipline and persistence to master the forms.

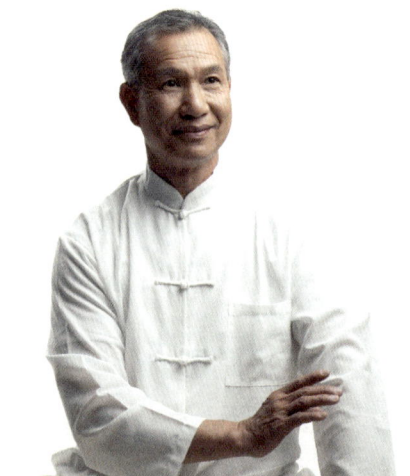

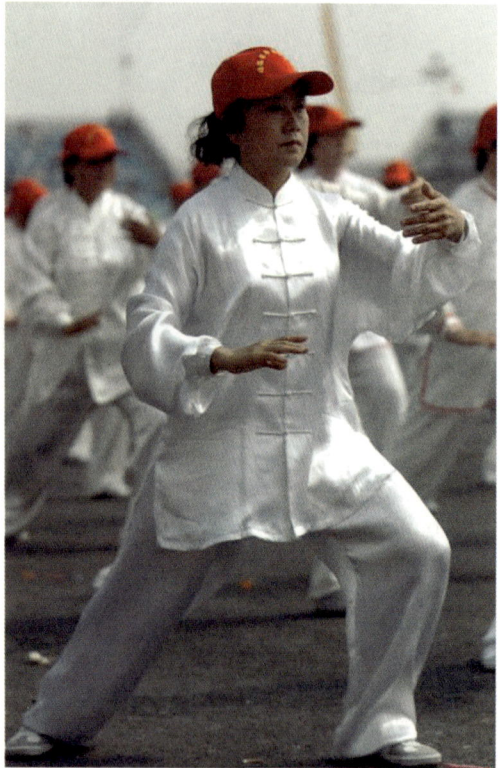

It is highly recommended that you learn tai ji quan from a qualified instructor. A DVD can help you get a rough idea about the basic movements and the sequence. But tai ji quan is not dancing or modeling, where the external form is most important. You need an experienced instructor to guide you through the internal process as well as the external movements.

You need to practice on a regular basis. Find a quiet place with fresh air (like a garden or the woods). Get yourself familiar with the movements first, and then you will start to feel the subtle difference it makes on your body.

With a calm mind, guide your movements consciously, breathe slowly, deeply and naturally. Your movements should be stable, constant, gentle, and fluent. By learning to do the movements slowly but consistently, your body can be trained to follow the subtle instructions of the brain. This is the way coordination between your body and mind is gradually improved. A friend of mine who has practiced tai ji quan for five years once fell down from a riding bicycle and to her surprise, she was not hurt at all. At the instant she fell down, her body naturally folded into the best position to avoid a head injury. The ability to adjust to the environment is a higher level of vitality and leads to a greater state of health.

Tai ji is both yin and yang: moving and still, hard and gentle, backward and forward, flexible and firm. Practicing tai ji quan can boost your qi and harmonize the yin and yang of your body. Practicing tai ji quan can make you feel refreshed, relaxed, and help you feel the joy of being alive. Tai ji is a door into the world of rediscovering your own body and how it relates to the world outside. It is for everyone.

Qi gong

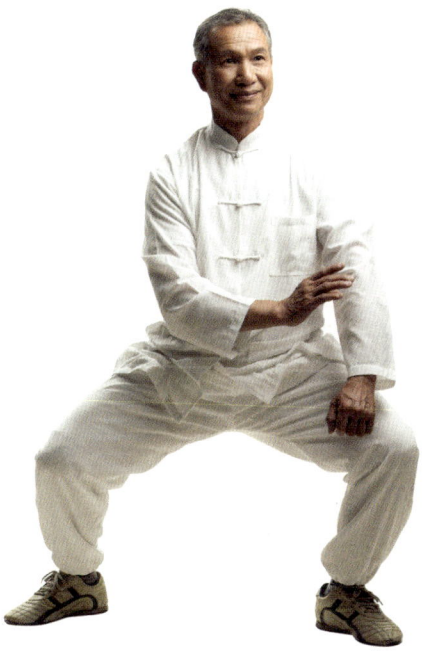

Qi gong is divided into moving and still qi gong. Moving qi gong is practiced by coordinating body movements with breath and mind. Tai ji quan can be considered as one kind of moving qi gong but they are not exactly the same. Static qi gong focuses mostly on control and coordination of breath and mind, which is more difficult for beginners. Moving qi gong, which is often mistaken for tai ji, is what most people have seen before. Qi gong is not magic, nor is it mere exercise. It is an important element of Chinese medicine. During the Spring and Autumn (770-476 BC) or Warring States (475-221 BC) period, a monograph on qi gong entitled *Xíng Qì Yù Pèi Míng* appeared. This text, possibly over 2500 years old, was the first written reference to qi gong.

From the perspective of Chinese medical theory and practice, qi gong can supplement qi, strengthen

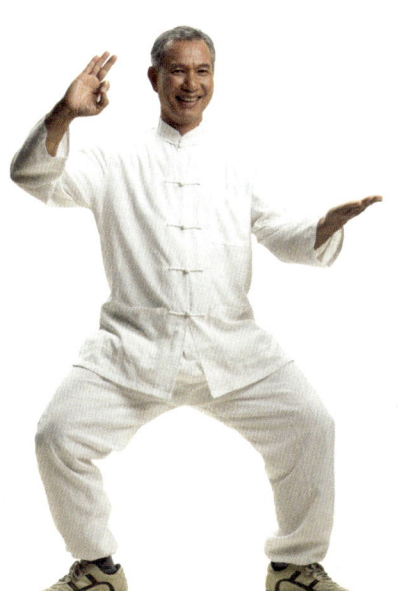
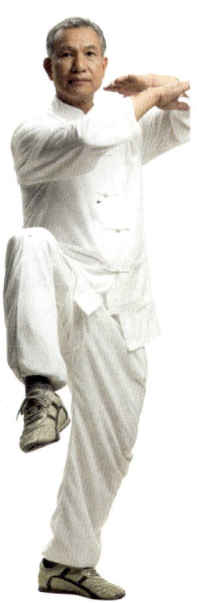
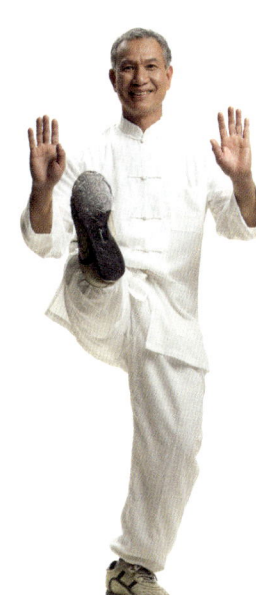

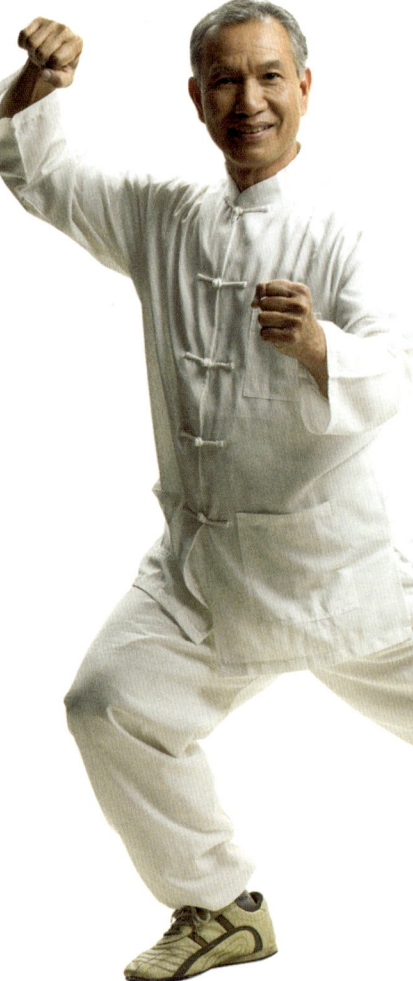

the body, harmonize yin and yang, regulate qi and blood, smooth the flow in the channels, and calm down the mind. It can relieve symptoms related to diabetes, lower blood sugar, improve the function of the pancreas, correct metabolic disorders, and prevent complications.

Personally, I first experienced a qi gong treatment when I was about 15 years old. It was performed to treat pain that was diagnosed as dampness and qi deficiency. I had severe pains in my knees that got worse before it rained. I couldn't sleep because the pain was so bad. The treatment was performed by a folk qi gong practitioner in my community. It was amazing and I still remember it to this day. I felt her power like a magnetic force during the treatment and afterwards a shoe-shaped wet mark appeared where I was standing (the floor was dry and I was wearing boots!). My knees haven't been painful since.

However, it is more difficult to locate a real qi gong practitioner than to find a tai ji practitioner because qi gong is not easy to learn, practice, or evaluate. Scientists are still exploring specific methods to study qi gong and some are showing prospects (please see the section on research).

The key to practicing qi gong is the regulation and coordination of body, mind, and breath. You also must choose the type suitable for your condition. In most cases you will need an instructor.

Here we have quoted a qi gong routine especially for the disease *xiao ke* (diabetes), which originated from the *General Treatise on Causes and Manifestations of All Diseases* (*Zhū Bìng Yuán Hóu Lùn*) written by Chao Yuan-fang in 610 A.D. It is easy to learn and safe to practice, and is mostly for those with a strong thirst and frequent urination. There are three steps. It can be practiced 2-3 times per day.

Step 1 Moving qi while lying down

Loosen your clothes, unbuckle your belt. Lie comfortably on your back. Stretch your lower back by pressing your sacrum against the bed or floor and arching your back. Place your hands naturally on both sides of your body. Close your eyes gently. Touch your upper palate (the gum line on the inside of the mouth) with your tongue. Breathe through the nose deeply, slowly, evenly, and quietly five times. Make sure your lower abdomen moves with the rhythm of breathing and you don't breathe shallowly with your chest. Keep your lower back slightly arched during the five breaths.

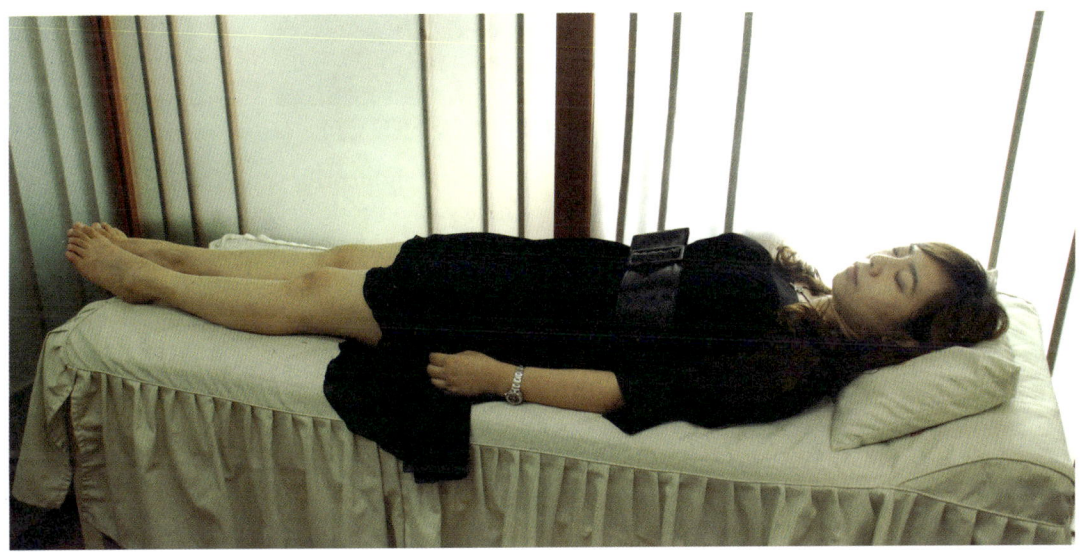

Step 2 Twirling tongue and swallowing saliva

Twirl your tongue clockwise between the teeth from top to bottom and from left to right 9 times then do it counter-clockwise between the teeth from up to down, from right to left another 9 times. Gargle without using any water and swallow slowly in several gulps the saliva produced. Lead the saliva down with your mind to lower *dān tián* (i.e. *guān yuán*, RN 4, about 3 inches below the belly button). Lie quietly for several minutes.

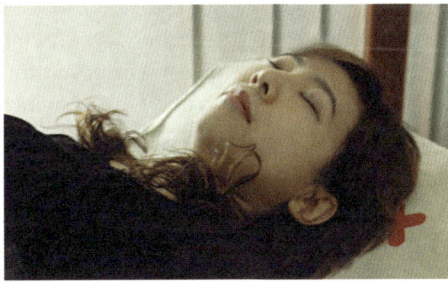

Step 3 Walking slowly

Go outdoors to a quiet, green, fresh environment (like a small lake with trees). Walk slowly in a happy and calm mood for about 120-1200 steps (depending on how much energy you have).

One needs guidance to practice qi gong. If you are obsessive while practicing, it may do more harm than good.

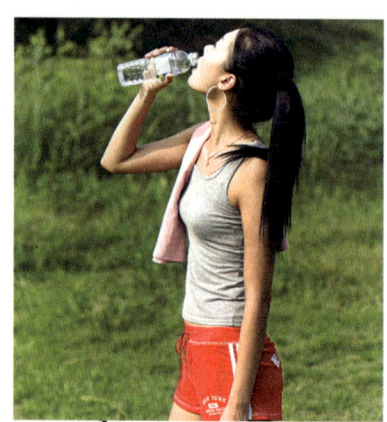

3. Translated Research

Over the past half century, the Chinese government has given a lot of support to the practice and study of its traditional medicine. Due to this support, thousands of clinical trials and research projects have been performed on the effect of acupuncture, Chinese medicinals, moxibustion, qi gong, and other modalities on different diseases. There is a wealth of scientific information that is largely unavailable in English. Below, and in the following chapters, we have summarized the results of some of the studies performed on patients with diabetes to show that not only are the results of Chinese medicine noticeable to the patient, but can be recorded by modern scientific techniques as well.

(1) A group of researchers conducted a literature review of the qi gong intervention studies published in English and Chinese since 1980. They were trying to determine the effectiveness of qi gong in the management of diabetes. The studies that were selected for review showed that qi gong had a positive impact on fasting and two hour oral glucose tolerance test results, blood glucose, triglycerides, and total cholesterol. There was no conclusive evidence that qi gong had an effect on body weight.

(2) A study compared the effects of normal walking and qi gong walking for 30 minutes after meals in ten diabetic patients with complications. The study found that both qi gong walking and normal walking reduced blood sugar faster after meals than doing no exercise. The significant finding, though, was that the patients who practiced qi gong walking maintained a lower pulse rate (79 beats per minute) than those who walked normally (95 beats per minute). This is an important finding for diabetic patients who have heart problems and need to be careful of their heart rate.

(3) Tai ji quan exercises were found to decrease blood glucose levels along with increasing regulatory T-cells and decreasing of cytotoxic T-cell populations in type II diabetic patients.

(4) A group of 39 ethnically Chinese adults

with at least one cardiovascular risk factor (hypertension, high cholesterol, smoking habit, or diabetes) joined a tai ji quan class for one hour three times a week for twelve weeks. The purpose of this study was to determine if tai ji could improve balance, muscle strength, endurance, and flexibility. At the beginning of the study all the patients fell below the 50th percentile of fitness in their age and gender groups. Improvement in all categories was evident after six weeks and further improvement after twelve, leading to the conclusion that tai ji practice could be of great benefit to the general health of the population.

(5) A twelve week study involving 14 adolescents with type 1 diabetes compared the effects of exercise three times a week to a control group who did not exercise. The study found that while exercise alone would not control type I diabetes, it did significantly increase endurance, improve body weight, and raise insulin sensitivity.

(6) A study selected 5,159 men from England who were previously free of disease in order to determine the effect of physical activity on the incidence of heart disease and type II diabetes. After an average 17-year follow-up, the authors concluded that the risk of developing type II diabetes decreased with increasing amounts of physical activity. Similar results were collected from the Finnish Diabetes Prevention Study conducted in 2000.

(7) A study done in 2000 in Beijing observed the effect of qi gong on 40 type II diabetic patients (5 years of diabetes on average). The intervention combined treatment from qi gong practitioners and the patient's own practice under guidance of a qi gong teacher. One year later 92% of the patients' blood plasma glucose had dropped below 7.8 mmol/L(140mg/dl) and patients said many of their symptoms had improved.

(8) A study in China compared the microcirculation (peripheral blood flow), blood sugar levels, and urine sugar levels before, during, and after qi gong treatment on diabetic mice compared with diabetic mice who received no qi gong and a control group of normal mice. Results showed that qi gong has an effect on microcirculation and urine sugar levels, but not on blood sugar levels in diabetic mice.

(9) Fifty type II diabetic patients practiced qi gong together 3 times a week (2h) and alone at home 1-2 times per day (30min). The researchers compared the blood sugar, symptoms, blood viscosity, and lipid levels before and after treatment. Results showed that blood sugar and lipid levels were significantly reduced. The general symptoms and any complications present also improved.

(10) A study done in Shanghai 1999 randomly divided 65 type II diabetic patients into a qi gong group and a control group. Both groups received a combination of western medication and Chinese medicinals. The qi gong group was asked to practice *bǔ shèn qiáng shēn* qi gong twice a day for three months. The results showed that the 2 hour plasma glucose and glycosylated hemoglobin levels dropped more significantly in the qi gong group. Insulin sensitivity index increases were also better in the qi gong group.

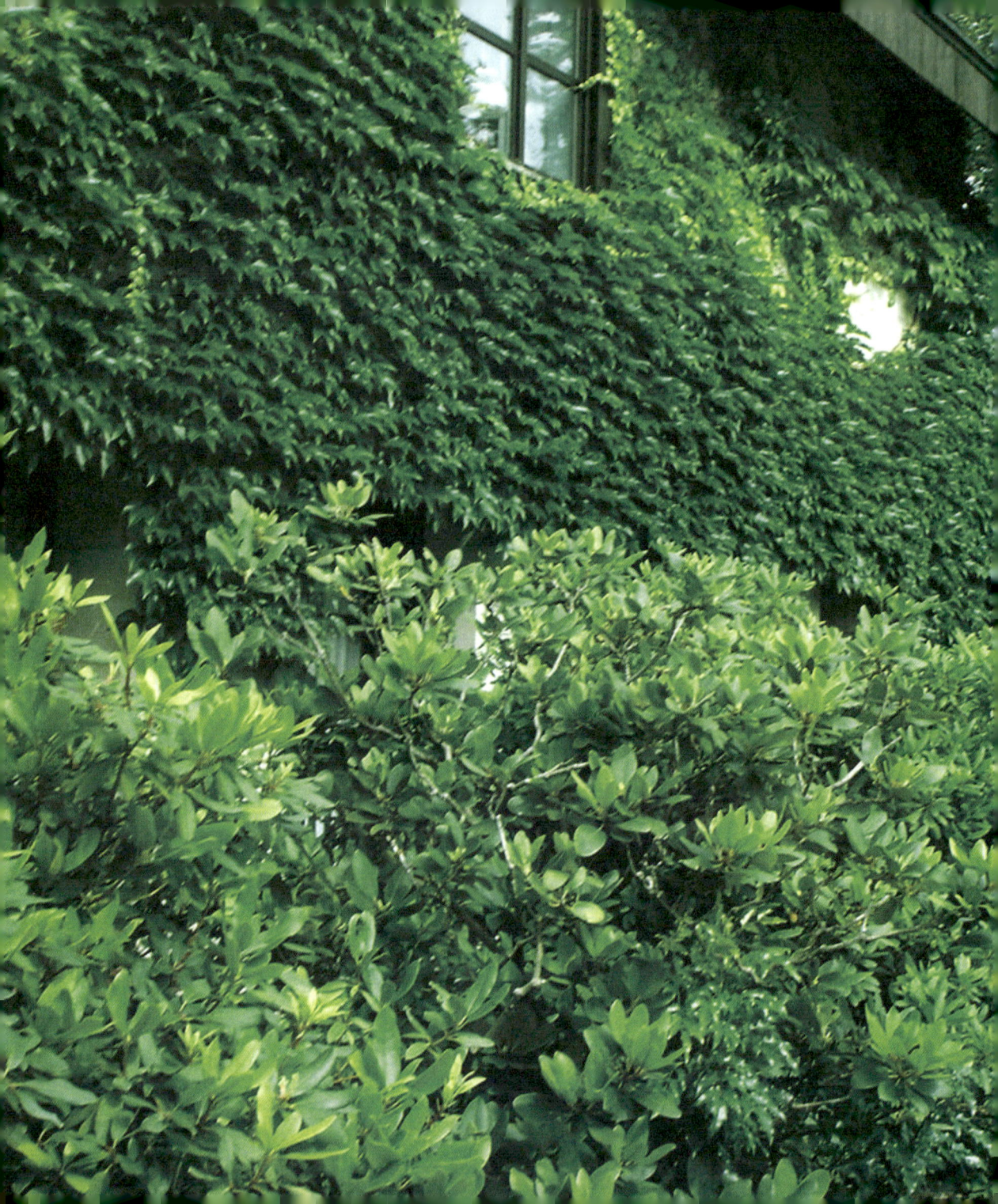

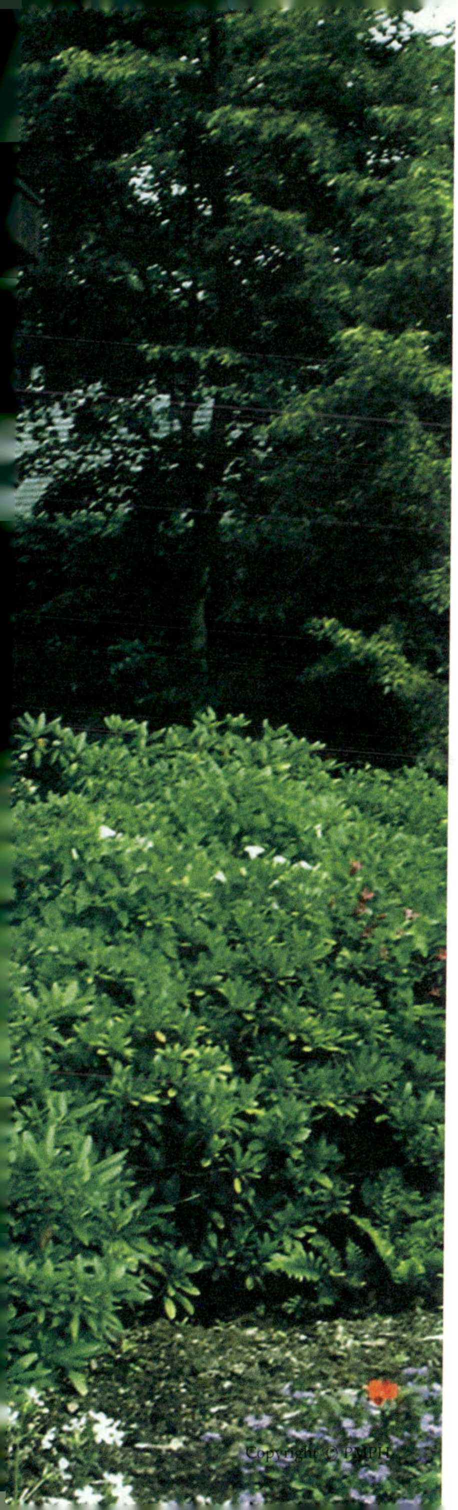

Chapter 4

How Does Chinese Medicine Manage Diabetes Mellitus?

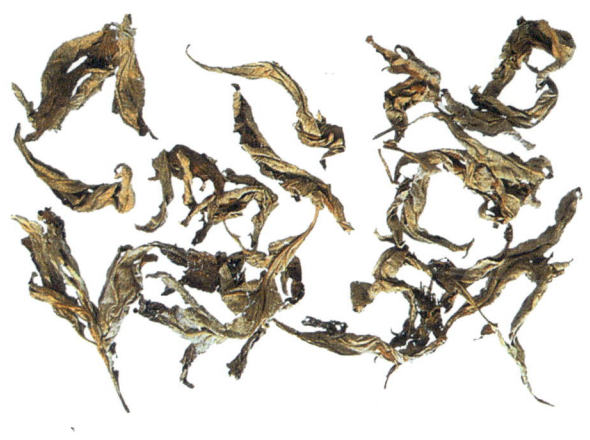

In the language of Chinese medicine, diabetes can be categorized into many patterns, the most frequent ones are as follows. They are:

- Deficiency of yin with internal heat
- Extreme heat due to yin deficiency
- Deficiency of qi and yin
- Deficiency of qi and yin with stasis
- Deficiency of yin and yang

Table 4-1 Five Common Patterns of Diabetes

Patterns	Symptoms	Treatment Principle
Deficiency of Yin with Internal Heat	strong thirst, dry mouth and throat, vexing hot feeling in the palms and soles, night sweating, a thin red tongue with little or no coating, and a fine rapid pulse	supplement yin
Extreme Heat Due to Yin Deficiency	severe thirst, increased appetite, dry mouth and throat, hot feeling in the palms and soles, frequent urination, dry stool, night sweating, a thin red tongue with a thin yellow coat, and a fine rapid pulse	supplement yin and clear heat
Deficiency of Qi and Yin	fatigue, weakness, sweating upon slight exertion, strong thirst, lassitude, dry mouth and throat, hot feeling in the palms and soles, sore and weak lower back and knees, frequent urination, dry stool, a light red tongue with little coating, and a fine rapid weak pulse	supplement qi and yin

Deficiency of Qi and Yin with Blood Stasis	symptoms from the above pattern plus: thirst that is worse at night, not drinking much water, dry scaly skin, menstrual disorders in women (clotted, dark-colored blood), fixed stabbing pains in the abdomen, a purple tonge or purple spotted tongue, and a fine wiry or rough pulse	supplement qi and yin, move blood and remove stasis
Deficiency of Yin and Yang	thirst, drinking lots of fluid, frequent urination at night, hot feeling in the palms and soles, fear of cold, lassitude, sore and cold and kness, weak limbs, spontaneous sweating, susceptibe to catching colds, abnormal bowel movements, an enlarged tongue with whitish or little coating, and a deep fine weak pulse	supplement yin and yang

The process of pattern differentiation is a highly intellectual, innovative, and individualized practice. Although in recent years, biomedicine has tried to achieve individualized treatment, it is fulfilled and practiced to the maximum extent in Chinese medicine. This is why when faced with different patients the Chinese medical practitioner will offer sometimes quite different prescriptions for each case. Pattern identification can only be accomplished by using sound judgment based on an interactive, humane interview between an experienced practitioner and a patient. The ability to do correct pattern identification is what defines a skilled doctor of Chinese medicine.

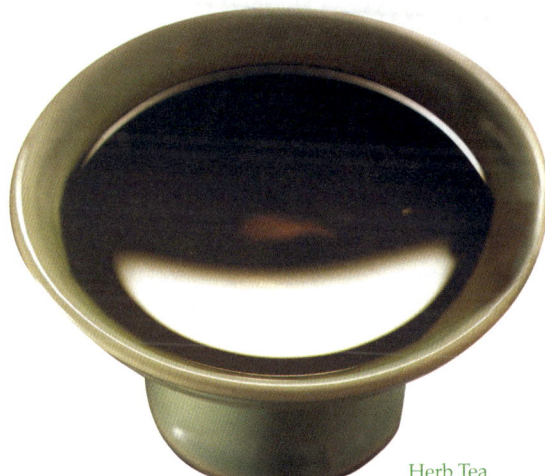

Herb Tea

Using pattern identification, treatment methods often vary. Herbal medication is the first choice in the treatment of diabetes and is administered orally or sometimes applied topically. Non-herbal medication includes acupuncture, moxibustion, tui na, etc. The exact prescription will consist of a detailed selection of herbs, their dosage and method of administration and an acupuncture point selection, manipulation techniques, and duration of treatment, all of which is based on the individual patient's pattern. Several treatment methods can be combined for the same patient to ensure comprehensive management.

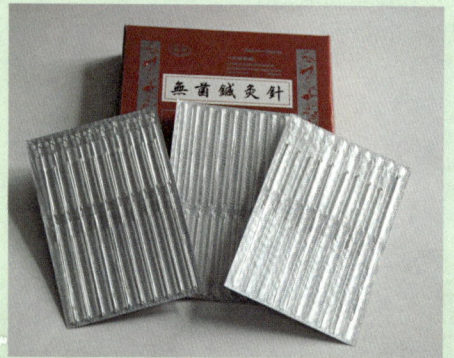

Acupuncture Needles

The use of modern biomedicine integrated with Chinese medicine has increased the scope of treatment available. With the help of modern technology, Chinese medicine has a better understanding of diabetes thanks to laboratory tests and biomedical diagnostic guidelines. Pattern identification becomes more accurate without losing its advantage of promoting the ability of human body to heal itself. Chinese medicine can provide numerous treatment methods for diabetes. The following sections will talk about the major ones.

Acupuncture and Moxibustion

1. What Is Acupuncture and Moxibustion?

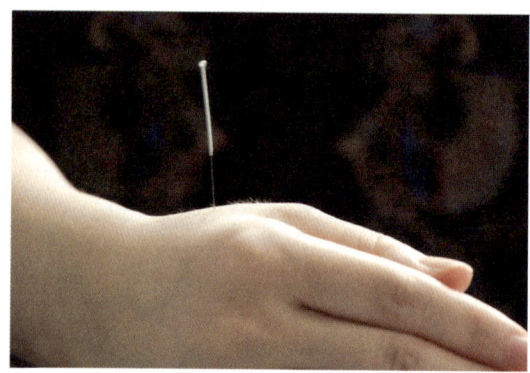

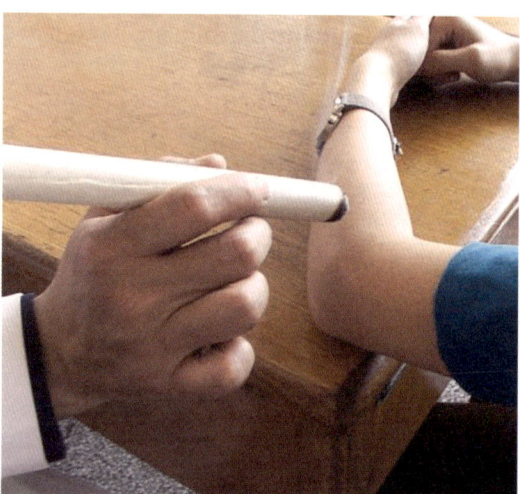

Zhen Jiu is the Chinese term that refers to acupuncture and moxibustion, the treatment methods that have been characteristic of Chinese medicine for thousands of years.

These days, acupuncture is everywhere. Visiting www.pubmed.gov and typing "acupuncture" in the search box, one can read hundreds of reports of research involved in the scientific exploration of this ancient art. Acupuncture and moxibustion have been proven effective in various diseases from cardiology to psychology. One reason these techniques are so popular is that they are absolutely safe when properly administered by a trained acupuncturist, although the thought of being needled can be unsettling to many first-time patients. For most people in the west, it is difficult to understand how a fine needle inserted into a part of the foot can relieve a headache, why a fetus's position can be reversed by needling a toe, or how puncturing a spot on the wrist could treat insomnia. All of these actions are easily explained in the language of Chinese medicine, but there are still many theories about how exactly it works in modern scientific terms.

In order to understand acupuncture, moxibustion, or channel theory, an understanding of Chinese medical theory is necessary.

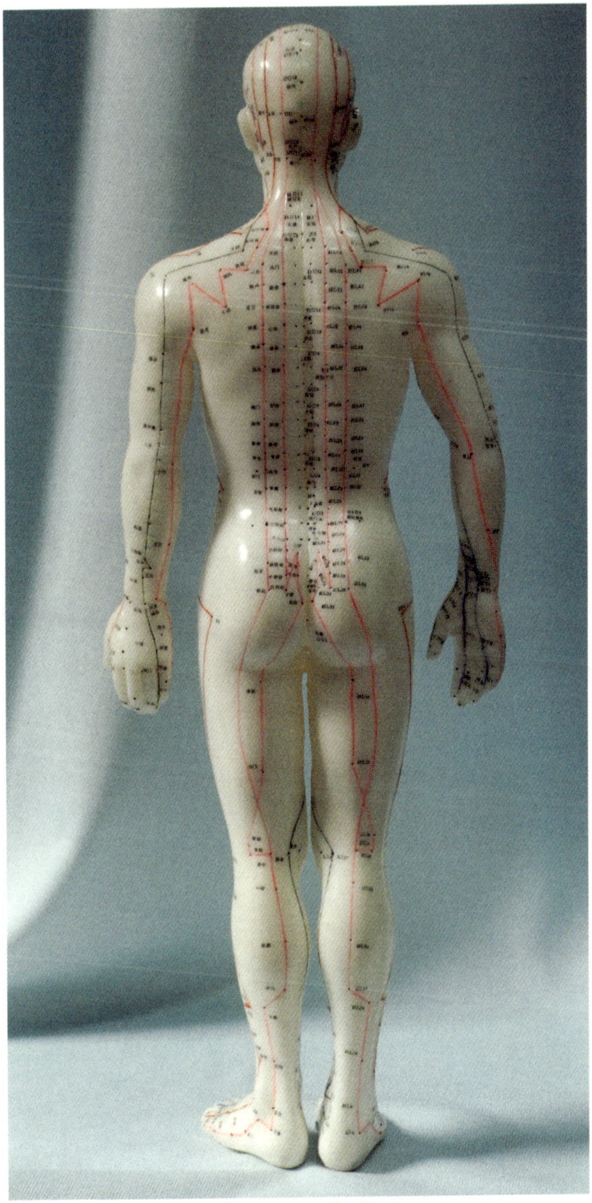

Channels on the Back

Channels & Collaterals
(Jīng luò)

In the theory of Chinese medicine, the human body is an organic whole and the internal organs, external surface, and extremeites are connected to each other by a network called the channels and collaterals (*jīng luò*). According to this theory, the channels and collaterals connect the internal organs with the external surface and extremities by transporting qi and blood. Analogy can be made between this network and the earth's water system. With big rivers as the main thoroughfares, and the tributaries as smaller branches, the whole planet is closely connected. Acupuncture and moxibustion are applied according to this system. By stimulating the points (*xué wèi*), or the gates of this network, the human body will be influenced, moving naturally towards healing. Acupuncture points are the openings of these channels and collaterals. Inserting needles into these points will stimulate or block the flow of qi and blood. When properly administered, the flow of qi and blood will be smoothed and organ functions will be restored. Weakness is strengthened while excess is reduced. Balance is restored and health is regained.

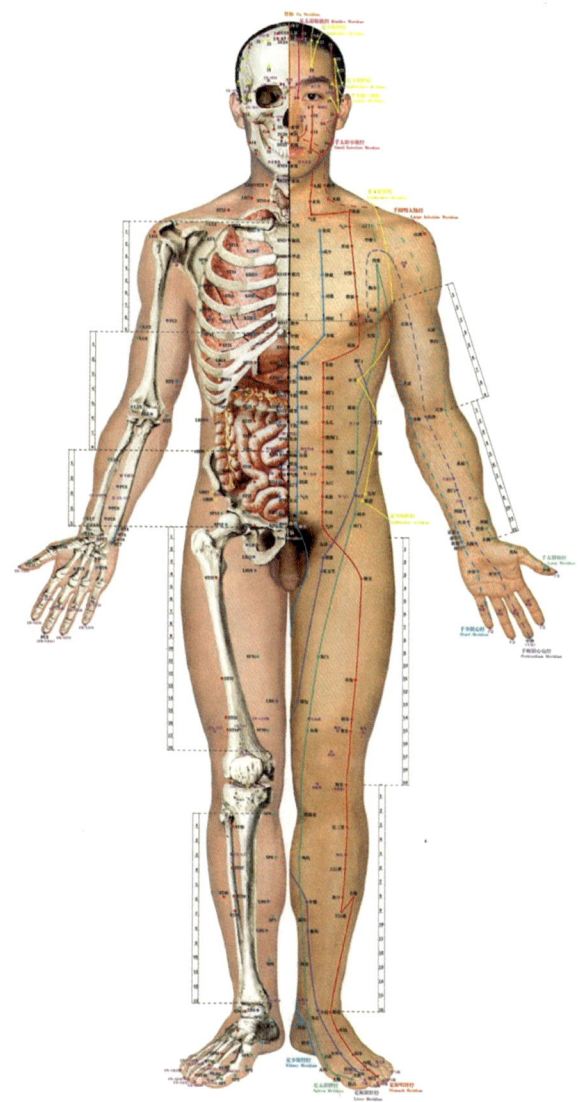

Acupuncture and moxibustion are best at regulating functional disorders. For example, acupuncture will help regulate the endocrine disorders in mild or intermediate diabetic patients and help the body regain its healing power. The disease progression can be delayed or even stopped. If administered on a regular basis, it is also possible to reverse structural damage by promoting functional recovery.

2. How Does Acupuncture Work?

The underlying mechanism is still being researched. There exist many theories as to how acupuncture may affect the human body, and each one can explain part of the picture. In studies of its pain-relieving effect, researchers found that acupuncture can block the impulse transmissions between the spinal cord and brain to stop pain by closing the nerve fibers that carry impulses. This is a common theory and often referred to as the gate control theory. Various other theories also attempt to answer the question from different angles. The theory of boosting immunity states that levels of important bodily substances such as white blood cells, antibodies, triglycerides, and gamma blovulins are raised during treatment and this stimulates the immune response. Another theory states that endorphins, which act to both stop pain and promote a sense of well-being, are stimulated through acupuncture. Neurotransmitter studies show that levels of seratonin and nor-adrenaline are altered during treatment. The circulatory theory involves the release of vasodilators, which cause blood vessels to constrict and dilate.

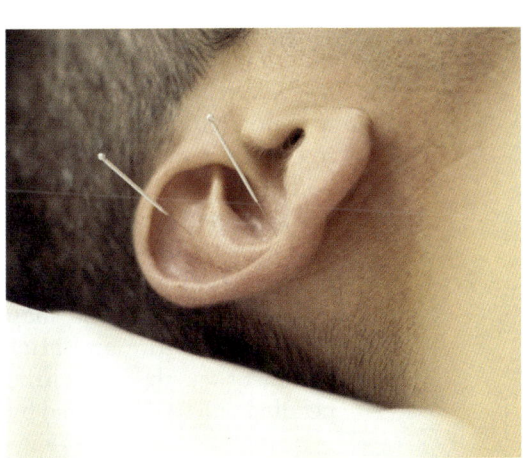

What we can conclude from these theories is that acupuncture acts on many targets. A synthesized drug has a definite target and expected effects, together with expected side-effects as well. The function of acupuncture is done in reverse by stimulating the body's power to regulate its own function and relieving localized symptoms. The relief of symptoms are only "side-effects" of the general changes going on at the root level.

Acupuncture needles

The most common acupuncture needles are called filiform needles, which are normally between 0.5 to 1.5 inches long (1.5–4.5cm), but can be up to 5 inches (15cm) depending on the location of the point to be needled and the size of the patient. The needles are usually made of stainless steel, but gold needles and silver needles are sometimes used. The needles are used on one patient and then disposed of in a medical "sharps" container.

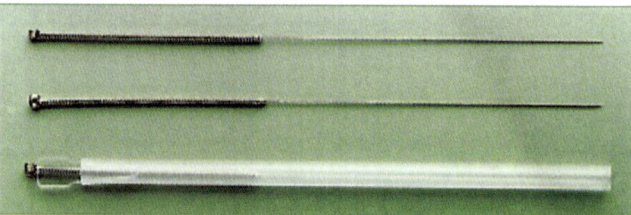

Acupuncture Needles

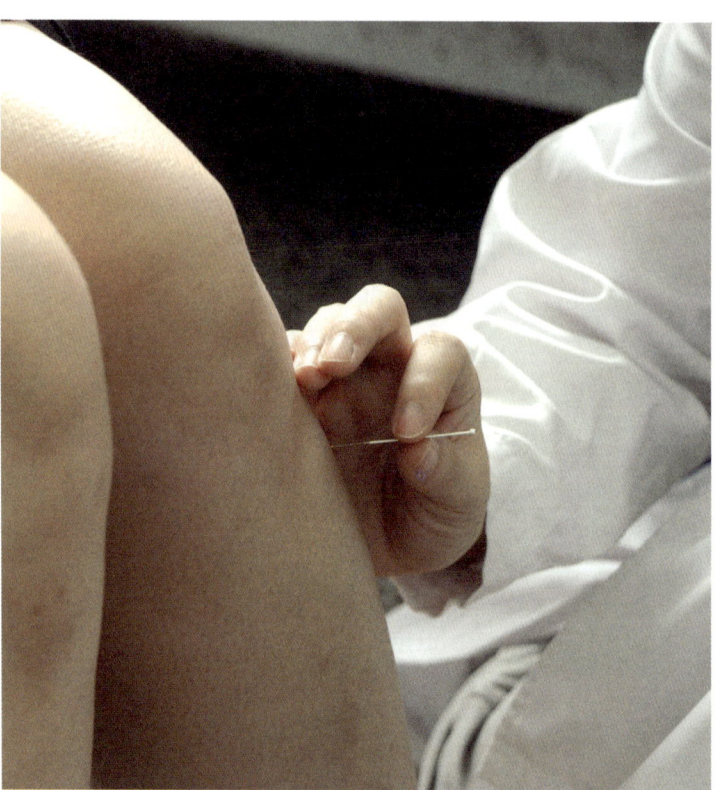

Acupuncture positions

Different positions are used based on the points selected. As long as the patient feels comfortable, any position is suitable.

Clean needling practice

Acupuncturists are required to take a course called the "Clean Needle Technique" to train them how to handle, insert, and remove needles so both patient and practitioner are protected from any kind of contamination. The acupuncturist will wash his or her hands thoroughly with soap and water before and after treatment, and the points to be needled will be disinfected by swabbing the point with a cotton swab dipped in 75% alcohol. Anything that punctures the skin will be sterile, and any other implements used in treatment will be thoroughly sanitized between patients. You don't need to worry about the possibility of contamination at all if you go to a licensed acupuncturist.

Electroacupuncture

Currently, it is common for practitioners to choose to use an electrical apparatus that allows an electrical impulse to be sent through the acupuncture needles to mimic constant manipulation. Practitioners are trained to operate the machines in the safest way and the amount of power sent through the needles is usually only a few microamperes. Electroacupuncture is commonly used for problems that require constant needle stimulation. The machine will allow the practitioner to do other work while the point is receiving stimulation. Originating in China, this technique is commonly used in many countries. The frequency and the amount of power used in electroacupuncture tends to vary to a great degree depending on the patient's condition and the practitioner's discretion.

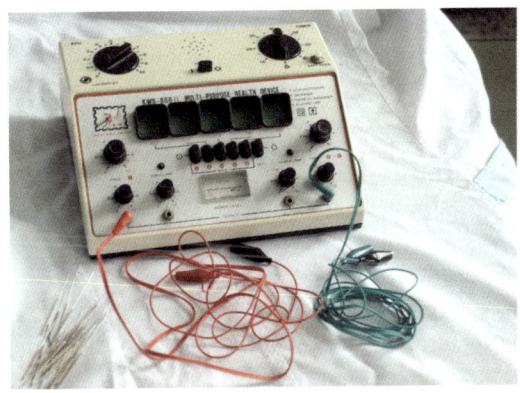
Electroacupuncture Apparatus

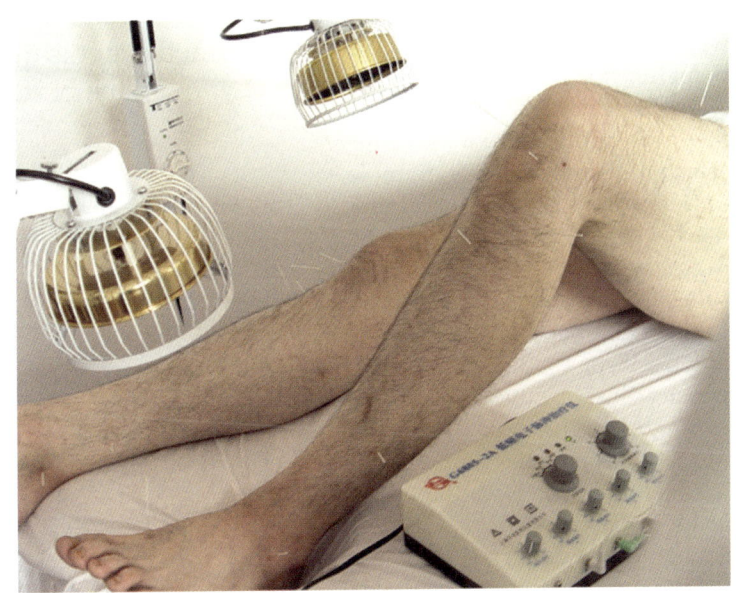
Electroacupuncture Treatment with Heat Lamps

Commonly used acupuncture points

There are hundreds of points on the human body, most of which are situated along 14 main channels. Some of the points are more commonly used than others. The points selected in the treatment of diabetes can vary greatly, according to the patterns, the patient, and the practitioner's experience. The final prescription of point selection depends on your specific condition and the practitioner's judgment.

The action of every point is to regulate yin and yang, the difference is in the exact way each point works. Some points work on the qi aspect, while others may work on the blood; some are warming, and others are cooling. Most point functions have not been verified by modern research, but for some of the more important points, some research has been done. For example, *yí shù* is an extra channel point commonly used in clinic. It has the effect of treating *xiao ke* (diabetes) according to *Invaluable Prescriptions for Emergencies* (*Bèi Jí Qiān Jīn Yào Fāng*, 700 A.D.) because it corresponds to the qi of the pancreas inside. Puncturing this point can regulate the qi of the pancreas. Modern research has found puncturing this point can lower blood sugar levels in diabetic rabbits. This effect is strengthened when it is combined with the important point *zú sān lǐ* (Stomach 36). This research provides evidence for the effects of acupuncture points.

We wish to stress that patients with diabetes must be very careful when receiving treatment with acupuncture and moxibustion since diabetic patients are more prone to infections. There are doctors that prefer not to use acupuncture and moxibustion when treating diabetic patients. Even without these cautions herbs are considered the best way to treat diabetes. But since acupuncture and moxibustion are effective for diabetes, you should take advantage of these therapies if possible. Be aware of your body and communicate with your practitioner. If you are cautious and the practitioner is qualified and responsible you will be perfectly safe.

Below are some photos and descriptions of commonly used points in the treatment of diabetes. Of course all patients are different, so not everyone will get all of these points. But since these are major points, everyone is likely to experience at least a couple of these points during the course of treatment.

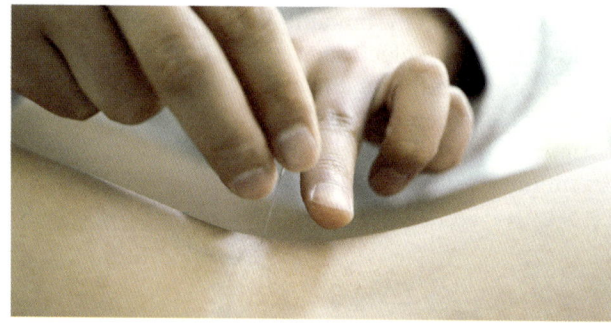

The locating of points is based on anatomical landmarks on the body surface, combined with bone measurement and finger measurement. So your measurement is different from others in length. It is also different in different parts of your body.

Zú sān lǐ (Stomach 36)

Arguably the most important point on the body, *zú sān lǐ*, which means "leg three mile", is the primary point used when the body's qi is weak. The name informs the practitioner that needling here will help the patient walk three more miles on their life journey. It is located on the stomach channel and can be used for any digestive disorder as well. Since the body's qi is largely produced by the digestive system, the importance of good digestion to health cannot be exaggerated.

Zú sān lǐ is located roughly one hand's breadth (4 fingers) from the bottom of the knee cap, on the outside of the leg. It is often somewhat sensitive when pressed.

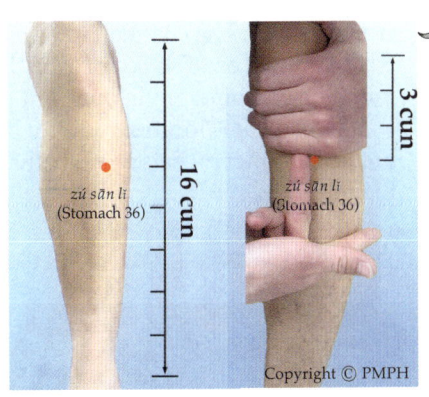

Pí shù (Bladder 20)

Located on the bladder channel *pí shù*, means "spleen transport" and is part of a group of "*shù*", or transport, points on the back, each of which corresponds to an internal organ. The organ which modern Chinese medicine translates as spleen is one of the central organs of digestion and qi production, and works closely with the stomach. *Pí shù* is used to harmonize weak digestive function and boost qi levels.

It is located roughly two finger widths from the spine on the level of the 11th thoracic vertebrae in the mid-back.

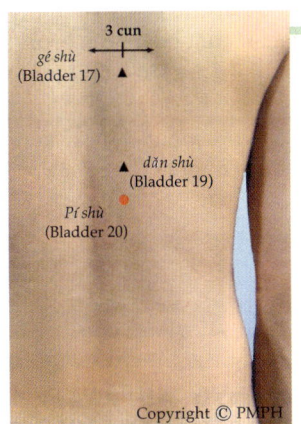

Yí shù (EX-B3)

Yí shù is another "*shù*" point on the back, but it does not lie on the bladder channel. "*Yí*" is pancreas in Chinese, and this point is considered an extra point. The function and importance of *yí shù* in diabetes was discussed above.

The point is located roughly two fingers from the spine on the level of the 8th thoracic vertebrae in the mid-back.

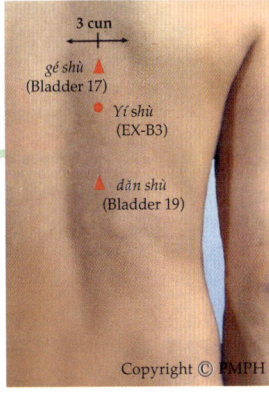

Guān yuán (Ren 4)

Located on a very yin portion of the body, the lower abdomen, *guān yuán* helps to nourish the yin of the liver and kidneys as well as strengthen qi. The channel it lies on, the Ren, is also known as "The Sea of Yin." It is a commonly used point for yin deficient patients.

Guān yuán is located roughly one hand's breadth (4 fingers) below the belly button on the mid-line.

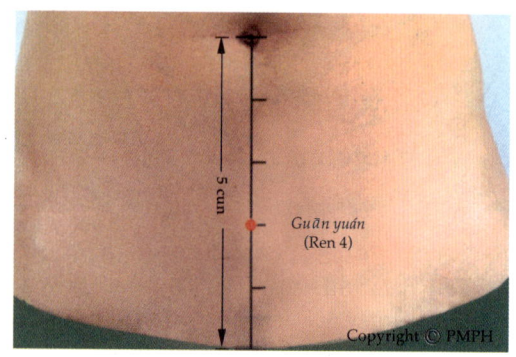

Shén mén (Heart 7)

Translated as "spirit gate", this point on the heart channel is commonly used to calm the mind. Emotional disturbances may affect the body in many ways, but it is often the heart that bears the brunt. *Shén mén* can soothe irritability and insomnia due to yin deficiency or ease anxiety due to qi deficiency.

The point is located on the wrist, inside the tendon that connects to the little finger.

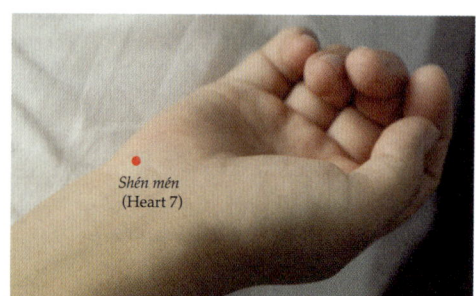

Sān yīn jiāo (Spleen 6)

Another point on a yin portion of the body, the inner lower leg, *sān yīn jiāo* is a very important point and used often for many disorders. Its name means "three yin intersection" and is a crossing point for the spleen, liver, and kidney channels, all of which are considered yin organs in Chinese medicine. Its location at an important intersection helps it to regulate organ function in many ways. It can both boost deficiency and move stagnation.

Sān yīn jiāo is located in the inner leg, roughly one hand's breadth (4 fingers) above the ankle bone, in the muscle behind the shin bone.

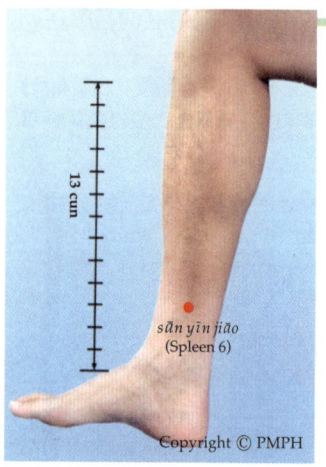

Case 4

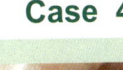

Mr. Wang, 56, was thirsty all the time. Over a few months time the symptoms got worse, so he visited a local doctor. He was diagnosed with pharyngitis and given antibiotics. But he didn't feel any better, and gradually his problem got worse. Again he visited a doctor and this time his lab results showed high blood glucose levels and the doctors suspected diabetes. Wanting to avoid tak-

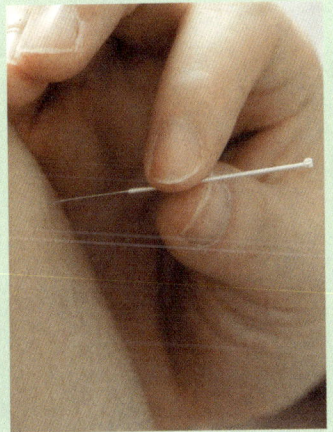

ing medication, Mr. Wang decided to give Chinese medicine a try. He visited the clinic every day for a 30 minute acupuncture session. After a month, he went back to the doctor for more lab tests. Happily, his blood sugar was within normal range. Perhaps more importantly to Mr. Wang, his severe thirst was gone. In a follow-up visit six months later, he reported no relapse.

Moxibustion

Moxibustion is the application of heat using a small bundle of tightly bound herbs that are burnt over targeted acupuncture points. By applying heat stimulation to certain points the practitioner can regulate the yin-yang balance of the internal organs to prevent disease, heal the body, and preserve health. It is another kind of external treatment method. The material used in moxibustion is usually made of artemesia leaves, commonly called mugwort. The Chinese medical classic *Miscellaneous Records of Famous Physicians* (*Míng Yī Bié Lù*) is a book on the pharmacology of herbs based on the legendary *Shen Nong's Herbal* (*Shén Nóng Běn Cǎo Jīng*). It states that artemesia leaves are bitter, slightly warm, without any toxicity, and are indicated for use in moxibustion to treat all types of diseases. Artemesia leaves, warm in nature, can promote the flow of qi and blood, remove dampness and cold, and dissolve masses and accumulations in order to cure illness, prevent disease and maintain health. Moxibustion has been used for thousands of years, longer even than stone needles, the ancient precursors to modern acupuncture needles. Like acupuncture, much research has been done on the effects of moxibustion on the body, but further exploration is needed to illustrate how exactly it works in scientific terms. Presently, it is widely used as an effective supplement to acupuncture treatment.

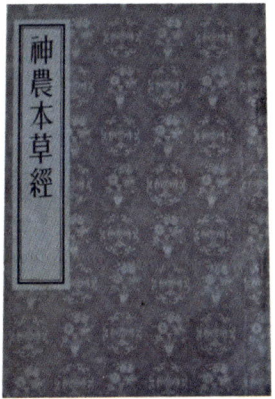

Shen Nong's Herbal
(*Shén Nóng Běn Cǎo Jīng*)

In the language of Chinese medicine, the major actions of moxibustion are to regulate yin and yang by supplementing yang, improve the circulation of qi and blood in the channels, help the body to fight invading pathogens, supplement qi and blood, and regulate the internal organs. These functions illustrate how moxibustion can prevent disease and delay ageing.

Types of moxibustion

The two main types of moxibustion are direct and indirect.

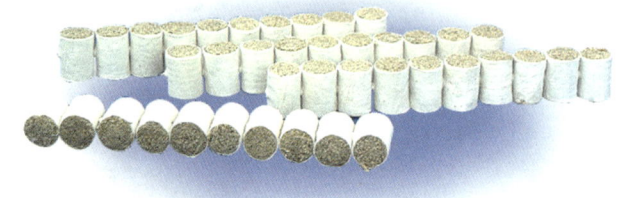

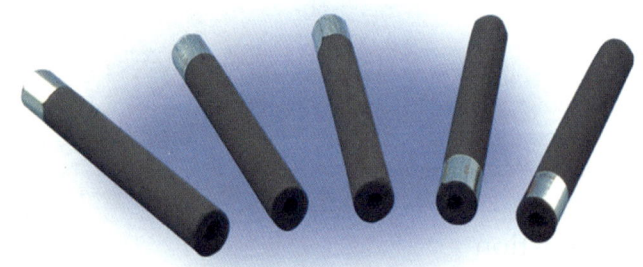

Direct moxibustion

Direct moxibustion uses what are called moxa cones. These are usually shaped to roughly half an inch (1.5cm) high, placed directly on acupuncture points, lit, and left in place until the cone is burnt out or until the sensation becomes painful. This is a strong form of treatment and can produce pain, blisters, and even scarring. Some Chinese traditions still deliberately induce scarring, which is believed to be most effective. This form of treatment is usually reserved for serious cases being treated by experienced practitioners.

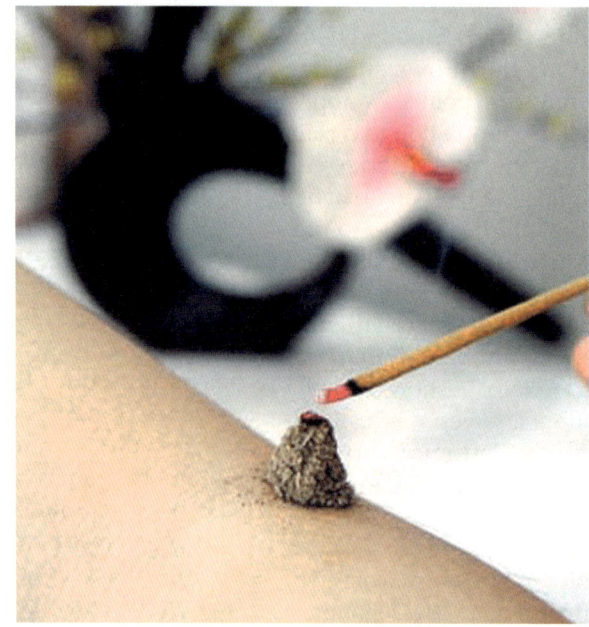

Indirect moxibustion

The second, more common form of moxibustion is indirect moxibustion. It involves either the use of a cigar-shaped moxa pole, or the burning of moxa cones on top of a layer of ginger, garlic, or salt. With a moxa pole, a practitioner holds the stick roughly 1.5 inches (4.5cm) above the skin and holds it in place until the skin becomes red or appears congested. When garlic, ginger, or salt is used with moxibustion, they provide a buffer from the heat of the moxa as well as adding their own properties to the therapeutic effect. These forms of treatment do not usually cause severe pain or leave any blisters or scars, though the skin may remain red for a while.

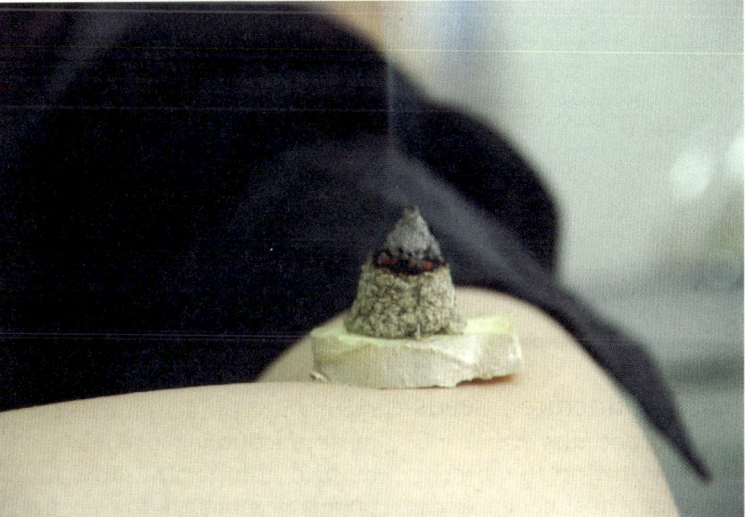

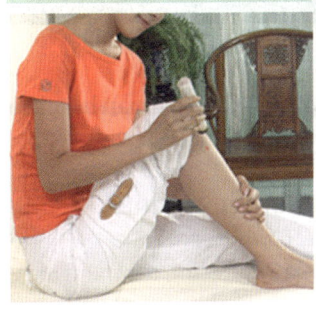

For people who have asthma or other respiratory problems, smokeless moxa can be used.

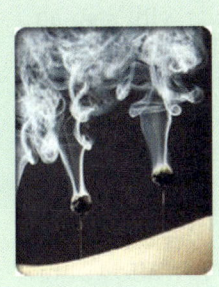

Practitioners also sometimes place the moxa cone on top of an acupuncture needle and burn it. If good ventilation is not available, heat can also be applied to points from an electrical source designed for the purpose as well.

Moxibustion is not for everyone. It is indicated mainly for patients suffering from cold or stagnation. It is not used on anyone diagnosed with too much heat. Since diabetics often have heat patterns, moxa is not used as often compared to other diseases. If there are isolated problems such as pain, injury, or digestive problems, moxa may be used. In addition, patients with diabetes must take extra care to avoid burns that may take a long time to heal.

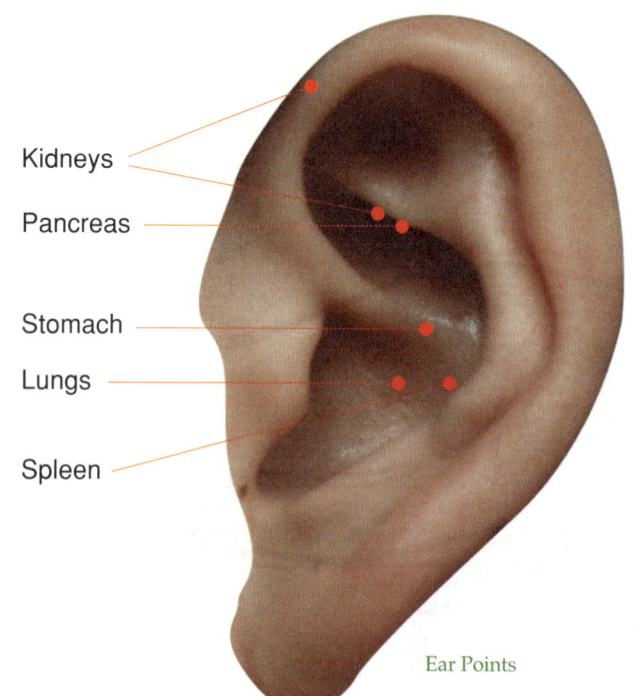

- Kidneys
- Pancreas
- Stomach
- Lungs
- Spleen

Ear Points

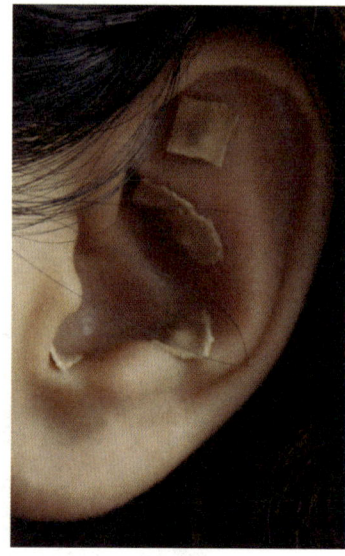

Ear Seed

Ear acupuncture / seeds

Placing needles in the ear is a new addition to Chinese medicine's treatment arsenal. Similar to reflexology, the ear represents a microsystem of the entire body. The shape of the ear is described by ear specialists as looking like a human fetus upside down, with the head as the lobe and the legs curled up to form the top. The entire human body with all its different parts and organs has been mapped out. Although there are specialists who mainly use ear acupuncture, most practitioners use it as a helpful adjunct therapy. A popular technique is to place a small seed, metal pellet, or tiny needle on an ear point and keep it in place with a small piece of tape. These objects will then provide a constant stimulation to the points chosen. Usually you will be instructed to press or rub each of these points several times a day for a few minutes. This convenient form of therapy allows for around the clock treatment. Normally the tape can be taken off in three or four days.

Other techniques

Though acupuncture and moxibustion are the main techniques used by practitioners of Chinese medicine, there are a variety of other techniques that may be used. These include but are not limited to cupping, gua sha, and plum-blossom needling. These techniques are used mainly for issues with pain and stagnation, though many practitioners use them in a wider scope.

We have decided not to include lengthy descriptions of

these techniques due to the fact that they are rarely used in the treatment of diabetes. The reason for this is that most of these techniques cause subcutaneous bleeding which results in slight bruising. Since it is often difficult for diabetic patients to heal from even small cuts, most practitioners will stay away from these techniques if a patient is diabetic.

Cautions and contraindications for treatment with acupuncture and moxibustion

Acupuncture and its adjunct modalities are an incredibly safe kind of therapy. However, there are certain times when great care must be taken in treatment and even times where treatment should not be administered. Fortunately for the patient, the scope of techniques available to the practitioner of Chinese medicine is very wide. If one treatment avenue is blocked, there will probably be another that is open and available.

Diabetic patients who are at an advanced stage should be especially careful with any kind of manual therapy that might cause damage to the skin in any way. Bleeding, burns, bruises, etc. are much more serious in the advanced stage of diabetes than in a healthy person. If you are at this stage, please inform your practitioner before treatment so the proper precautions can be taken.

The following are some other cautions and contraindications for treatment with acupuncture, moxibustion, or other techniques.

1 Any acute metabolic disorder like diabetic ketoacidosis or hyperosmolar coma is contraindicated for acupuncture and moxibustion.
2 Diabetic skin infections or ulcers are contraindicated for acupuncture and moxibustion. The patient can still receive treatment on other places of the body, but only if great care is taken.
3 Extreme hunger, fatigue and mental stress are not indicated for acupuncture and moxibustion.
4 Pregnant women can be treated, but the practitioner must be very cautious.
5 History of fainting during acupuncture treatments.
6 Chronic or severe diabetic patients are suggested to combine acupuncture and moxibustion with biomedical drug therapy.
7 Acupuncture and moxibustion treatment must go together with dietary restriction and life style management.

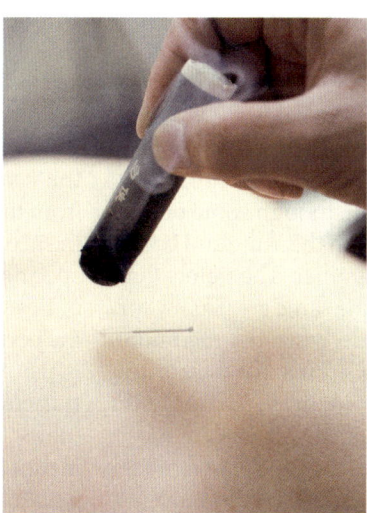

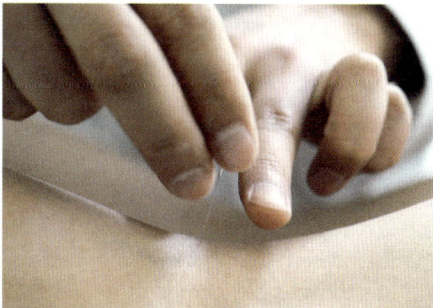

3. What Will My Treatment Program Be Like?

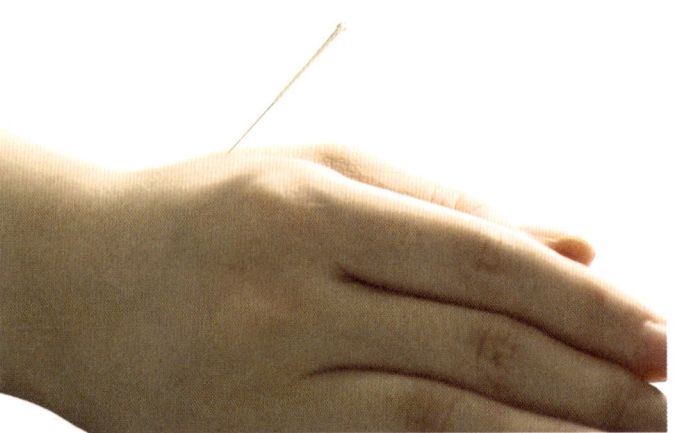
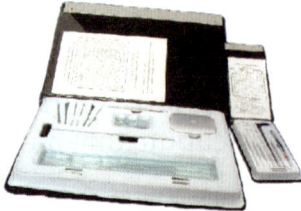
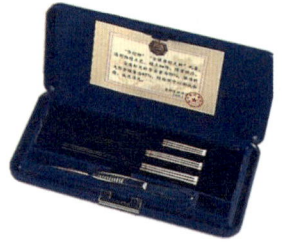

Needles

What can I expect during an acupuncture treatment?

After collecting detailed information (symptoms, signs, environment, tongue inspection, and pulse taking) the Chinese medical practitioner will identify the pattern of disharmonies present. Based on this pattern identification, an optimal treatment protocol will be drawn up according to theories of Chinese medicine.

The practitioner will then decide which modality (needles, moxa, cupping, etc.) to use during the present treatment. Usually needling is performed and often one or more additional treatment modalities are used. The number and location of the needles is decided by the acupuncturist and will probably vary from treatment to treatment, though some points will remain the same and begin to feel familiar. The points that remain the same are usually for your underlying root condition, while the points that change frequently are often to deal with whatever symptoms are most serious at the time of treatment. The amount of needles is not set and can be as few as 2 or 3 or as many as 30, but usually it is around 10 to 15. The needles are mainly placed on the abdomen, back and limbs, with points on the scalp and face also used from time to time. The depth of the needles is determined by the specific points since the amount of flesh is different throughout the body. The length of needles is also decided by point the acupuncturist chooses and normally is between 0.5 and 1.5 inches (1.5–4.5cm).

The needles are inserted quickly at an angle of 15 to 90 degrees in relation to the skin's surface. When an experienced acupuncturist inserts the needles, you normally will not feel any pain. The sensation is at most like being bitten by an ant. Acupuncture needles are much finer than the hypodermic needles used in hospitals. But most importantly, trained acupuncturists can insert the needles quickly and correctly without causing unnecessary discomfort.

Once the needle has been inserted there are a variety of techniques like raising, thrusting, twirling, plucking and scraping, which strenghten the stimulation and sensation. The technique used will depend on the disease that is being treated. The patient is supposed to get a specific sensation called "*dé qì*".

Dé qì is a sensation specific to acupuncture treatment and literally means "obtaining the qi". The exact feeling varies with each individual patient. It is usually not pain but a unique sensation of soreness, heaviness, distension, or radiation in some direction. It is generally believed that the stronger the *dé qì* sensation is, the more effective the acupuncture treatment will be. After a few treatments, patients usually start to enjoy this sensation because it is pleasant and they know the good results it brings.

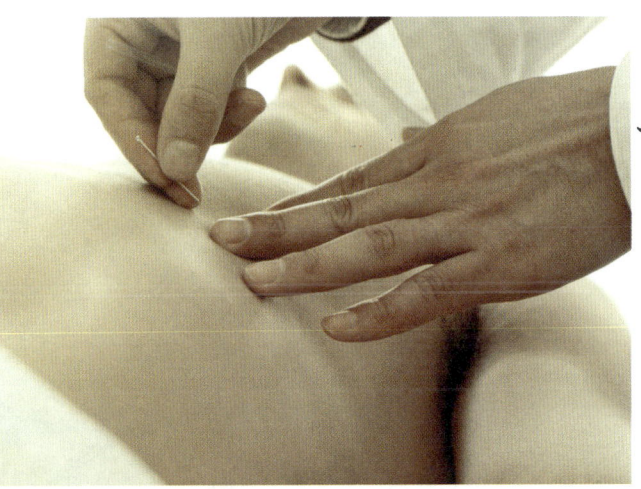

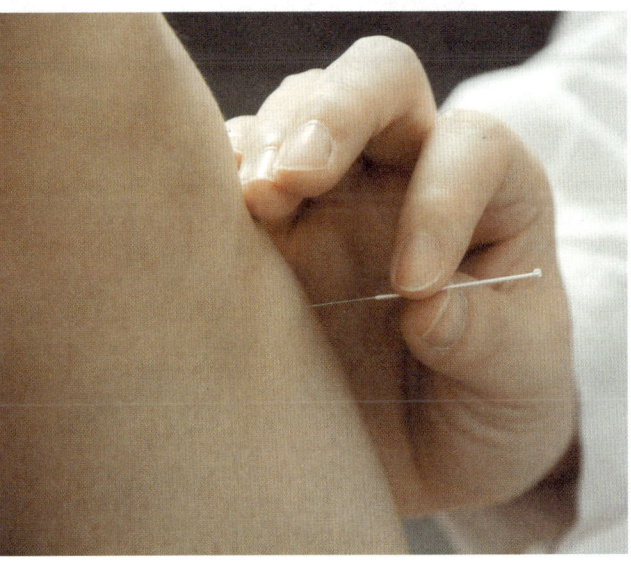

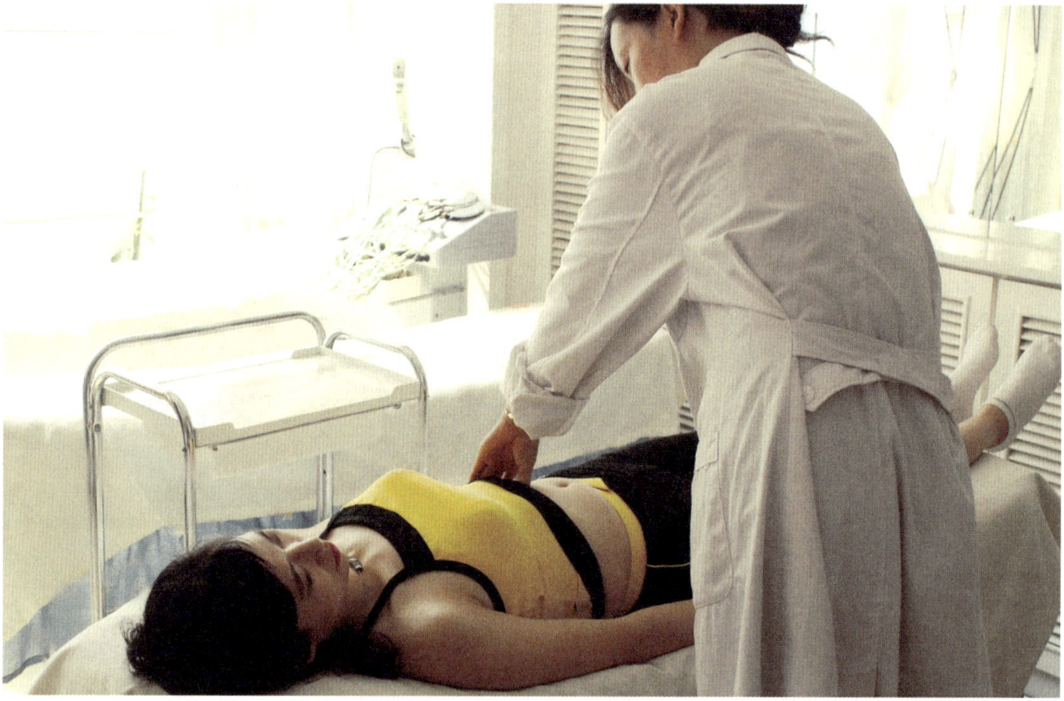

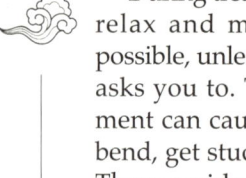

During treatment, it is best to relax and move as little as possible, unless the practitioner asks you to. Too much movement can cause the needles to bend, get stuck, or even break. These accidents are very rare, but if anything happens, stay calm and let the practitioner remove the needles immediately.

After the needles are inserted, the patient is usually left to relax for about 20–40 minutes. Other techniques such as moxa or cupping can be performed before or after needling, depending on the practitioner. After the needles are removed, get up slowly and carefully. There is normally no bleeding during or after acupuncture treatment. If bleeding occurs, it will only be a few drops due to the breakage of small capillaries. Bruising is also very rare, but sometimes happens due to subcutaneous bleeding also from broken capillaries.

After treatment, you will probably feel relaxed and energized. Some of your symptoms may disappear instantly. You may sleep better, have a more regulated appetite, feel less pain, or experience less anxiety. In care cases people might be over responsive to the treatment. This usually happens when a patient is extremely hungry, weak, nervous, or the stimulation and *dé qì* sensation is too strong. The patient might feel nauseous and possibly even vomit, develop a very pale complexion, feel weak, sweat excessively, or even faint. If this happens, the acupuncturist will take out all the needles immediately and let the patient lie down and rest for a while. Normally the patient will recover quickly. If the patient still feels unwell, a few points may be needled that will help relieve the patient's symptoms.

It is advised to be in the best condition possible when you have your acupuncture treatments. Don't come for your acupuncture treatment when you are very hungry or just after a big meal, and try to be rested. Get the most out of your treatment by being extra careful of your general health the day before and after treatment.

Treatment course and expectations

A typical treatment course will be 2-3 visits to the acupuncture clinic per week for 3-6 weeks. After this the practitioner and patient will re-evaluate and decide on future treatment. Since diabetes is a chronic disease, treatment will often take several months.

Even though most patients begin to feel some relief after the first few treatments, Chinese medical treatment is working on a very deep level and to effect lasting change, ample time must be given. The journey to health with Chinese medicine is like everything else in the natural world, there will be ups and downs, times of rapid growth and times of hibernation. With commitment and good communication between practitioner and patient, the journey can be life changing.

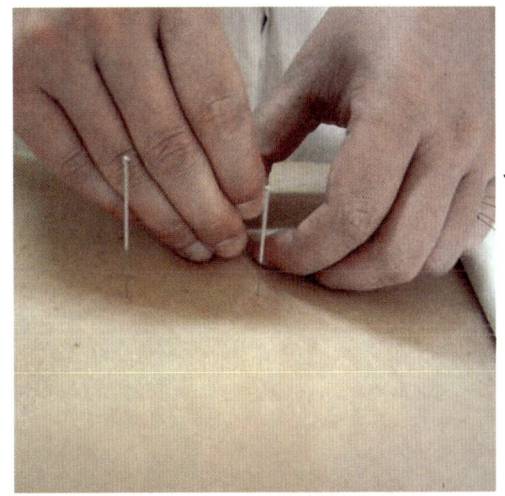

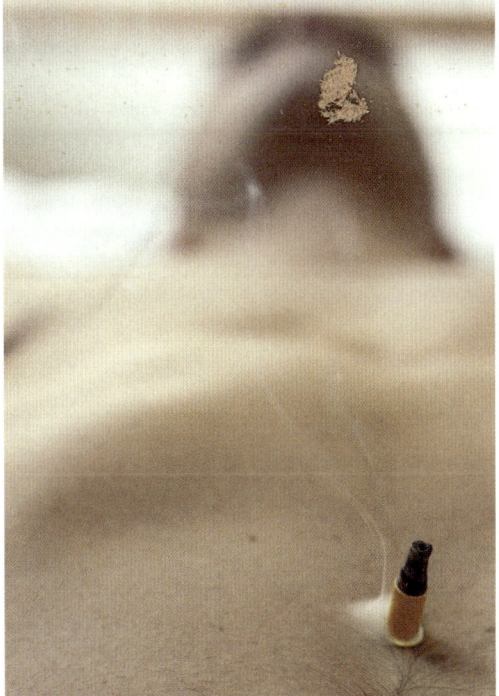

4. Translated Research

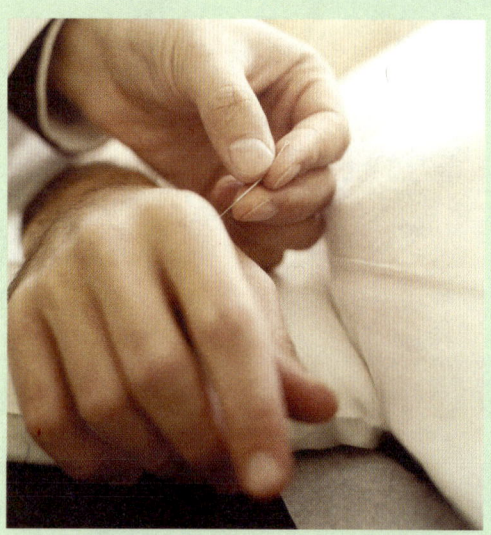

(1) A study in Kunming, China, in 1996 among a group of 42 patients with non-insulin dependent diabetes mellitus, randomly assigned them into an acupuncture group, a moxibustion group and an acupuncture plus moxibustion group. Results showed that in all three groups the clinical symptoms all improved markedly after treatment. Furthermore, after treatment the levels of fasting blood-glucose, saccharified hemoglobin, and glucose in the urine were significantly different before and after treatment. The therapeutic effect in the acupuncture plus moxibustion group was the best.

(2) A study in Liaoning, China, in 2006 among a group of 60 patients with Type II diabetes showed that by using acupuncture along with Chinese herbal medicine over a course of 45 days, their blood sugar was lowered by an average of 1.740 mmol/L (31.32 mg/dl) over a control group that received only Chinese herbal medicine.

(3) A study in Nanjing, China, in 1999 among a group of 46 patients with non-insulin dependent diabetes showed that by receiving acupuncture over a course of 1 month, their blood sugar was lowered by an average of 3.30 mmol/L (59.4 mg/dl) over a control group of healthy volunteers.

(4) A study in Henan, China, in 2002 divided a group of 80 patients with diabetes mellitus randomly into an acupuncture treatment group (A), an exercise therapy group (B), an acupuncture plus exercise therapy group (C), and a control group (D) treated with dietary advice and oral administration of hypoglycemic agents. The results showed that acupuncture and proper exercise can significantly decrease blood sugar and insulin and improve lipid metabolism, showing the possibilities available for treatment of type II diabetes. Insulin levels in groups A, B, and C decreased significantly after treatment as compared with those in the control group. Levels in the combined acupuncture-exercise group C were lower than those in group A and B. And the blood lipid levels in groups A, B, and C decreased somewhat as compared with levels before treatment.

(5) A study in Hangzhou, China, in 2001 among a group of 65 patients with Type II diabetes showed that by using acupuncture along with dietary restrictions over a course of 30 days, their

blood sugar was lowered by an average of 1.97 mmol/L (35.46 mg/dl) over a control group that received only a placebo (combined vitamins).

(6) A study in Hubei, China, in 2006 among a group of 60 diabetes mellitus patients with gastroparesis showed that by using moxibustion over ginger along with biomedical and Chinese herbal medicine treatment over a course of 30 days, their clinical symptoms of gastroparesis such as vomiting and anorexia were significantly relieved compared with a control group that received only biomedicine and Chinese herbal medicine.

(7) A study in Shandong, China, in 1996 among a group of 45 patients with diabetes mellitus showed that by using acupuncture along with biomedical treatment over a course of 100 days, their serum corticosteroid levels, which can be an indicator of blood sugar levels, were lowered by an average of 114.8 ug/L over a control group that received only biomedicine.

(8) A study was done in Tianjin, China, where 72 cases of diabetic gastroparesis (DGP) were randomly divided into a treatment group and a control group. The treatment group was treated with a needling method for harmonizing the digestion, with the points *qū chí* (LI 11), *hé gǔ* (LI 4), *zhōng wǎn* (RN 12), *Zú sān lǐ* (ST 36), *fēng lóng* (ST 40), *yīn líng quán* (SP 9), *sān yīn jiāo* (SP 6), *xuè hǎi* (SP 10), and *dì jī* (SP 8) selcted. Treatment was given twice a day for 10 days. The control group was treated with an oral administration of Motilium 10mg, 3 times each day, 30min before meals. The total effective rate (symptom relief index more than 20%) of 91.7% in the acupuncture group was better than 77.8% in the control group.

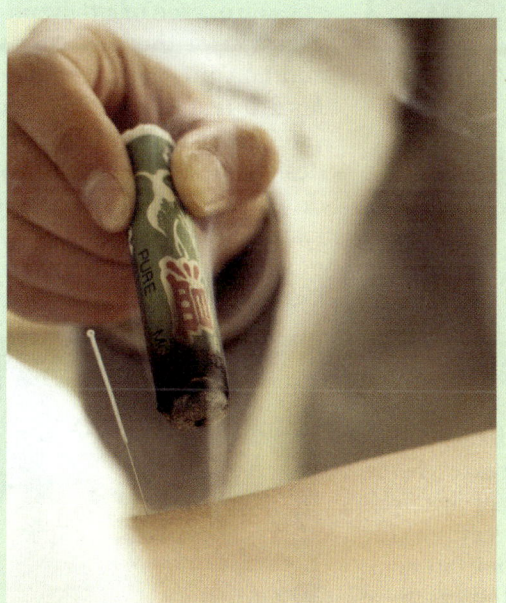

(9) This study was done in Kunming, China. 100 diabetes cases were randomly assigned into two groups: treatment group (60 cases) and control group (40 cases). The two groups both received conventional biomedical therapy. The treatment group also received Chinese medicinals and acupuncture treatments focused on moving blood and removing stagnation. After treatment, symptom relief and electromyelogram changes were both significantly better in the treatment group than in the control group.

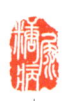

Chinese Medicinals

1. What Are Chinese Medicinals?

Introduction

The phrase "Chinese medicinal" refers to substances that occurs naturally in nature which comes from plant, animal, or mineral sources. These substances can be prepared in a variety of ways so that they can be used by the body. Chinese medicinals can be drunk, eaten, inhaled, or applied to the skin. They can regulate the body's qi, blood, yin, yang, and expel pathogens as well. There are over 3000 different substances listed in ancient pharmacology books, though only about 400 or so are commonly used. In fact, any natural substance can be used in Chinese medicine, but it will be called a Chinese medicinal only when it is used according to the theories of Chinese medicine.

In chronic metabolic disorders such as diabetes, Chinese medicinals can be used to relieve symptoms, manage the course, and improve the patient's quality of life.

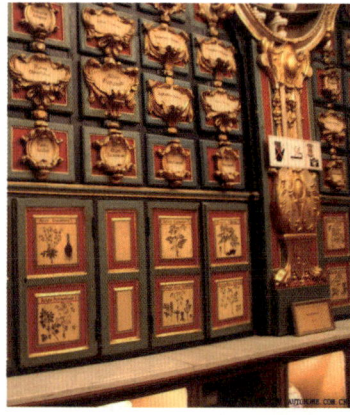

Mechanism of Chinese medicinals

The underlying idea between how Chinese medicinals work is fundamentally different than that behind biomedical pharmaceuticals. A pharmaceutical is a finely crafted and intensely focused creation. Years, sometimes decades, of research goes before any drug is released on the market. The scientists strive to isolate the exact chemical or combination of chemicals that can cause a very specific change in some bodily functions. The change elicited by these drugs is often effective at relieving symptoms, but does not usually restore the damaged body part or function whose breakdown was responsible for the symptoms in the first place. For example, antibiotics will kill invading bacteria, but will not strengthen the body against further invasions; or a pain killer may relieve the aching joints of an arthritis patient, but it will not stop or even retard the progression of the disease. In addition, it is not uncommon for a drug to cause unwanted side-effects in addition to its desired actions. Biomedical drugs may damage the nervous system, the digestive system, or most commonly the liver or kidneys.

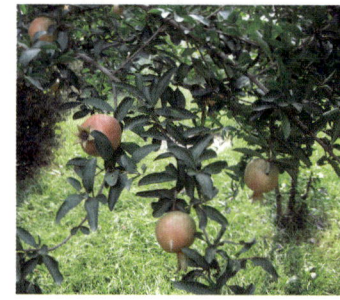

In Chinese medicine, as mentioned above, the idea is to restore the body's innate ability to remain in a state of health. In severe cases, long term treatment is necessary to provide constant support to the body, but usually patients who start treatment with Chinese medicine are able to stop treatment after their symptoms have been brought under control. Treatment is able to be stopped because the medicine used was helping to restore the body's damaged functions, not just substitute for them. Then these patients gladly use the principles of Chinese medicine throughout their lives to maintain health, only visiting an acupuncturist or herbalist to take care of any minor health problems that may crop up.

To a doctor of Chinese medicine, side effects are a sign of improper treatment, either due to faulty diagnosis, or inappropriate treatment methods. A properly constructed herbal formula will exactly match the patient's internal patterns and will not cause any other kind of imbalance. What is weak will be strengthened, what is too strong will be reigned in, leaving no room for other problems to develop due to the ingredients of the prescription. It is commonly thought that because Chinese medicnals include the whole biological substance (as opposed to an artificially isolated biologically active constituent), the naturally occurring ingredients that make up the harmonious living organism help to buffer the body from side effects. Here is an anology. Taking vitamin pills can help to quickly supplement nutrients you need. Yet they cannot replace food (a mixture of necessary nutrients and "unnecessary" substances) for the long-term maintenance of health. So is the case with synthesized drugs. Many of them are extracted or synthesized from natural plants. They are effective and helpful, but they cannot replace natural herbs (a mixture of effective ingredients and "ineffective" ingredients) for the long-term treatment of chronic diseases.

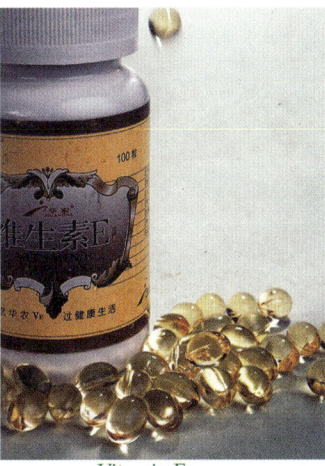
Vitamin E

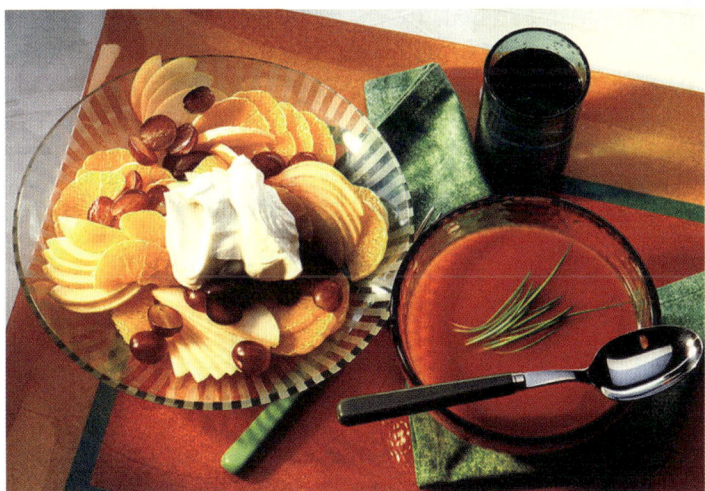

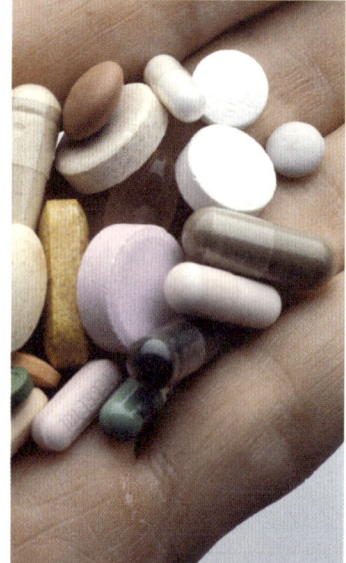
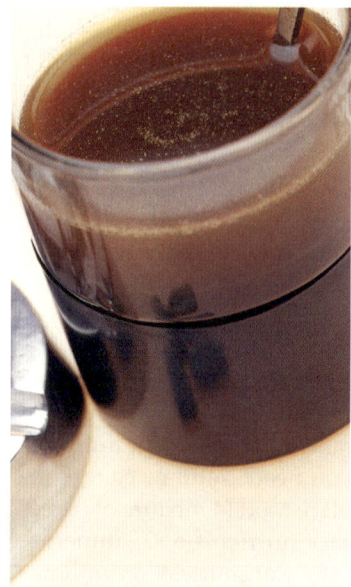
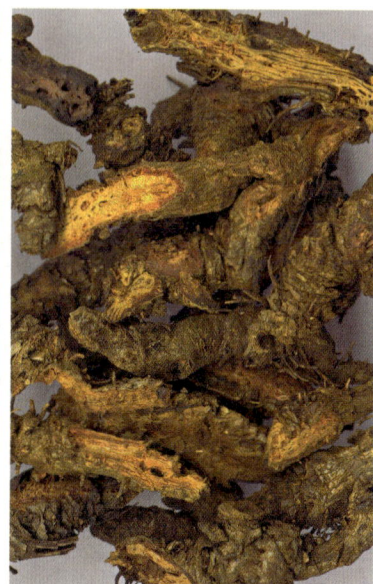

huáng lián (Rhizoma Coptidis)

Another mechanism that makes Chinese medicinals safe is that they are counterbalanced within the formula. As an example, medicinals that take out excess heat from the body are considered cold, and can damage the digestive system. Therefore, in formulas that are made to treat excess heat, a few medicinals that promote and strengthen digestion are added. If the patient has weak digestion to begin with, even more ingredients are reserved for that purpose. This kind of treatment is much more than simply anti-symptomatic. Each prescription must be a balanced entity, which perfectly compliments the patient's condition. When used properly, Chinese medicinals are safe and effective. This takes experience and active involvement by the practitioner. Sound and individualized diagnosis is made based on the patient's present condition to ensure efficacy and safety.

Classification of Medicinals

Every herb has unique properties including its nature (warm, cool, or neutral), taste (sour, bitter, sweet, acrid, salty), and function. Proper selection of medicinals is the key to avoiding side-effects. As they say, "One man's meat is another's poison".

A medicinal gets its property from a combination of factors including how it tastes, and how it affects the body. For example, *huáng lián* (Rhizoma Coptidis) is defined as cold since it tastes bitter and it relieves heat syndromes with symptoms like thirst, mouth ulcers, constipation, and a yellowish tongue coating, all of which taken together indicate excessive heat.

The selection of the medicinal is made according to the pattern identified. If the diabetic patient presents with signs of qi deficiency like shortness of breath, fatigue, lack of energy, weak pulse, and a pale tongue with thin whitish coating, medicinals that can supplement qi will be added. If signs of yin deficiency are obvious such as emaciation, feeling hot in the afternoon, night sweats, irritability, a fine pulse, and a thin tongue with little coating, medicinals that supplement yin will be administered. In clinical practice, practitioners of Chinese medicine gradually form a number of basic prescriptions (usually called formulas in Chinese medicine) that fit the common patterns seen in each disease. These formulas will be modified according to each specific case.

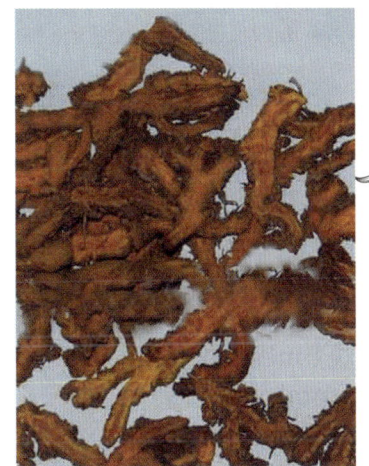

huáng lián (Rhizoma Coptidis)

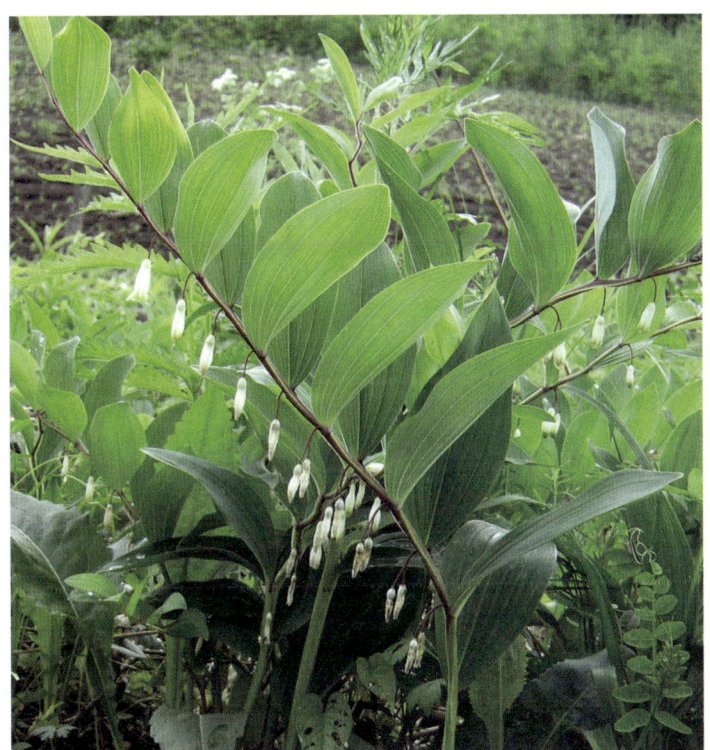

yù zhú

Modern research scientists have been investigating the mechanism behind these medicinals in the treatment of diabetes. In a recent review it was shown that the effects of medicinals commonly used in the treatment of diabetes have several different mechanisms depending on the substance. For example, the major component of *dì huáng* (Radix Rehmanniae) can stimulate the pancreas to secrete insulin. *Gǒu qǐ zǐ* (Fructus Lycii, recently popularized as "Gou Qi Berries") can protect the pancreas and improve its function as well. *Huáng qí* (Astragalus or Radix Astragali) extracts can increase the body's sensitivity to insulin and prevent insulin resistance. Other herbs and formulas are also found to have effects through different avenues. Although a clearer and more complete picture of their mechanisms is needed, it is clear that Chinese medicinals can contribute to the successful management of diabetes in the clinic.

Chinese medicinals in common use

Chinese medicinals are very rarely used alone. But in order to construct a proper formula, the practitioner must be familiar with the properties of each individual herb. Since patients may present in any possible combination of patterns, any one of the thousands of medicial substances may show up in a patient's formula. But as we have seen, there are a few main patterns that typically present in a diabetes patient. And for each of these main patterns, there are certain medicinals that are most effective and therefore most commonly used. In addition, due to scientific research, some herbs are known to be more effective in the treatment of diabetes. Below are some brief descriptions of some of the most commonly used medicinals in the treatment of diabetes:

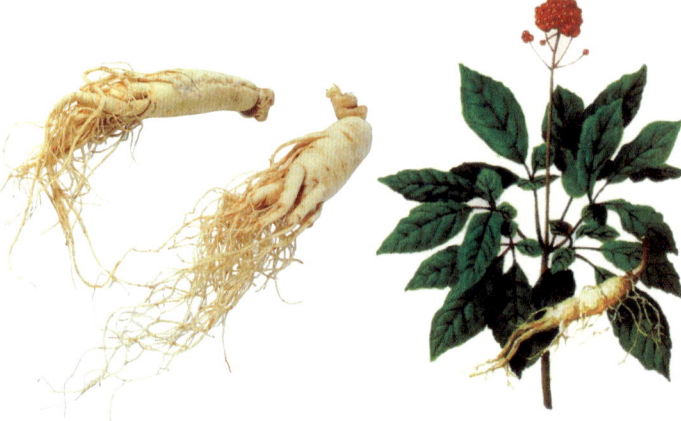

Rén shēn (Radix et Rhizoma Ginseng)

<Source> Ginseng root and rhizome

<Property> sweet, slightly bitter, warm

The famous Ginseng, the source of legends and currently found in energy drinks and vitamin supplements the world over, is an important herb for diabetics. Known as an "energy tonic", it does indeed build up the body's qi. But its secondary function, which makes it valuable in the treatment of diabetes, is to generate internal fluids, helping to stop thirst. Ginseng is powerful, but it is not for everyone. Those with too much heat will not see this root in their prescription, though it's American cousin *Xī Yáng Shēn*, who is slightly cool and has similar functions, may be used.

<Pharmacology studies>
Research shows that ginseng can lower blood sugar levels of normal and diabetic dogs, especially in the latter. Ginseng saponin (an active ingredient in ginseng) can significantly inhibit hyperglycemia for about 1-2 weeks. Clinical studies show that ginseng can not only relieve general symptoms like fatigue, thirst, and weakness, but also lowers blood and urine sugar levels.

Shēng (Shú) dì huáng (Radix Rehmanniae)

<Source> Chinese Foxglove Root – Raw or Steamed

<Property> sweet, bitter, cold (or slightly warm)

This root will be a dark, heavy, black chunk in your prescription packet, the quintessential yin substance. These herbs will replenish the yin and generate exhausted fluids in yin deficient diabetic patients. The fresh version is colder and used for those with more heat. The root becomes slightly warm when steamed. Both nourish yin, but the fresh root is said to clear heat from the blood.

<Pharmacology studies>

Both the fresh and steamed herb have the effect of lowering blood sugar levels and inhibiting hyperglycemia. The major effective component is rehmannin.

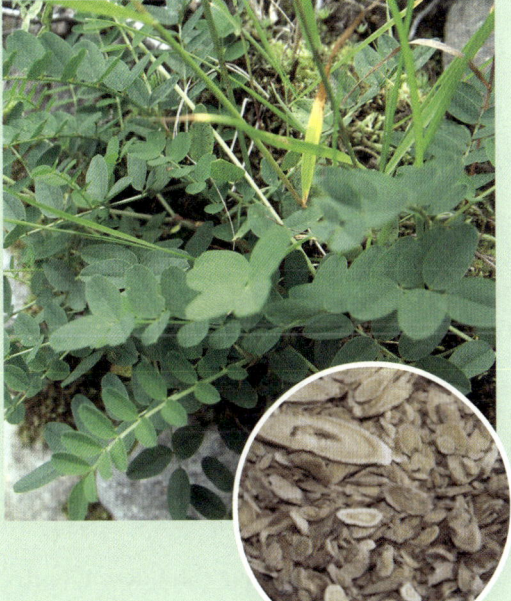

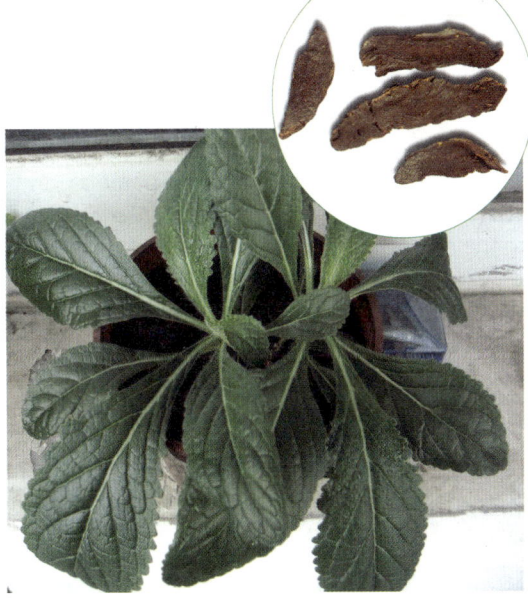

Huáng qí (Radix Astragali)

<Source> Astragalus root

<Property> sweet, slightly warm

Recently popularized for use during cold season for its immune building function, Astragalus is another qi tonic. It is not as warming as Ginseng, and its ability to stop sweating and keep the skin and muscles from stagnating make it useful in the treatment of diabetes mellitus.

<Pharmacology studies>

Research shows that *huáng qí* can improve heart muscle contraction, dilate coronary vessels, lower blood pressure, protect liver cells, and reduce blood sugar.

Xuán shēn (Radix Scrophulariae)

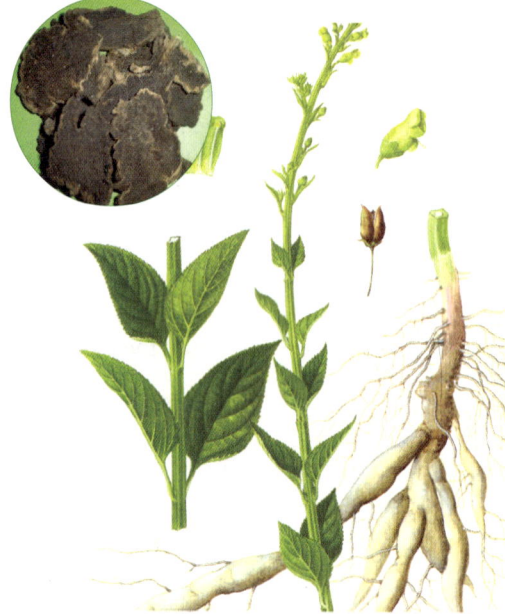

<Source> Scrophularia Root

<Property> bitter, sweet, salty, cold

The characters of this herb's name mean "Mysterious Root" and its function is similar to the raw Foxglove root mentioned above. It is also a heavy, dark substance that nourishes the yin and cools heat. Its Latin name Scrophulariae refers to the ancient function in both Western and Chinese herbology of treating swollen lymph nodes.

<Pharmacology studies>

According to modern research, it has the effect of lowering blood pressure and sugar levels.

Huáng jīng (Rhizoma Polygonati)

<Source> Siberian Solomon's Seal Rhizome

<Property> sweet, neutral

Huáng jīng comes from the genus Polygonati, which is the source of two important herbs to replenish yin. This herb is special because in addition to helping yin, it has a positive effect on the digestive system which is a major source of qi in Chinese medicine. *Huáng jīng* is also one of a very small number of herbs said to be able to "boost essence (*jīng*)" which is the bodily substance that when exhausted, means death.

<Pharmacology studies>

Its major components can lower blood lipids, sugar, and blood pressure levels and prevent atherosclerosis.

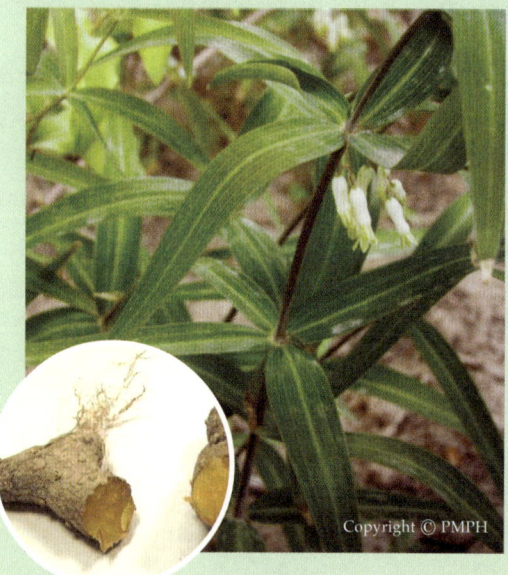

Dì gŭ pí (Cortex Lycii)

<Source> Wolfberry (Gŏu qĭ zĭ) Root Bark

<Property> sweet, bland, cold

From the same plant as Gou Qi Berries, this is the root bark and has a very different function. *Dì gŭ pí* is used in diabetes for its ability to cool the heat generated by a lack of yin. It is especially effective in cases of lung heat, which in Chinese medicine often manifests as excessive thirst.

<Pharmacology studies>

Dì gŭ pí can lower blood sugar and blood pressure levels. Rabbits given *dì gŭ pí* decoctions had a temporary rise in blood sugar levels that then quickly reduced for the next 4-8 hours.

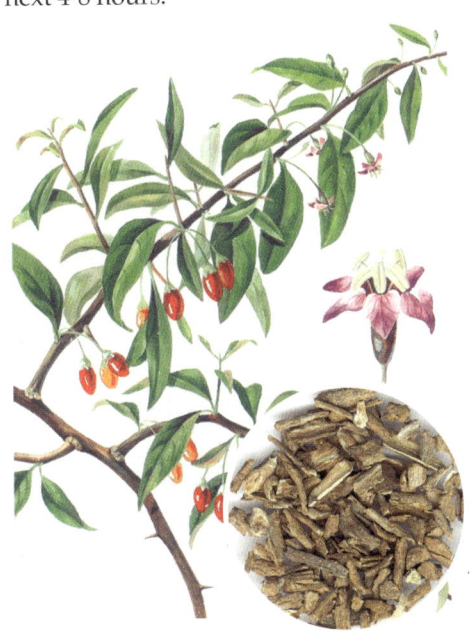

Gŏu qĭ zĭ (Fructus Lycii)

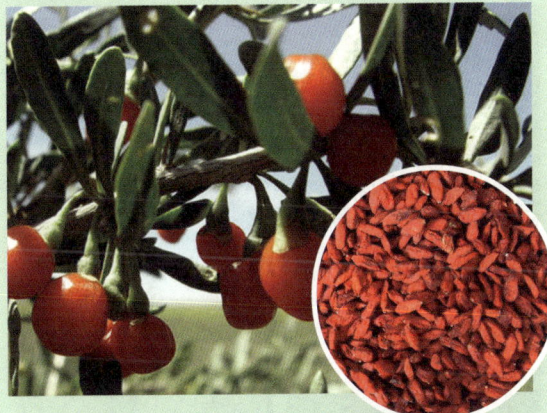

<Source> Wolfberry (Gŏu qĭ zĭ) Fruit

<Property> sweet, neutral

In the last year, this small red berry that when dried looks like a raisin, has become the health food world's golden child. Gou Qi Berries and juice are said to be a cure for almost any disease (even when covered with chocolate!). Though the Chinese medicine community sees this as a passing fad, these berries are nevertheless very valuable to herbalists. Seen as able to strengthen yin of the liver and kidney as well as protect and improve vision, this herb is often used in diabetes due to the regular clinical presentation of yin deficiency and the possibility of vision problems. *Gŏu qĭ zĭ* is another substance, along with *huáng jīng*, to belong to the elite group that can boost essence.

<Pharmacology studies>

Wolfberry has been shown to have the effect of lowering blood sugar, blood pressure, and lipid levels.

Gě gēn (Radix Puerariae Lobatae)

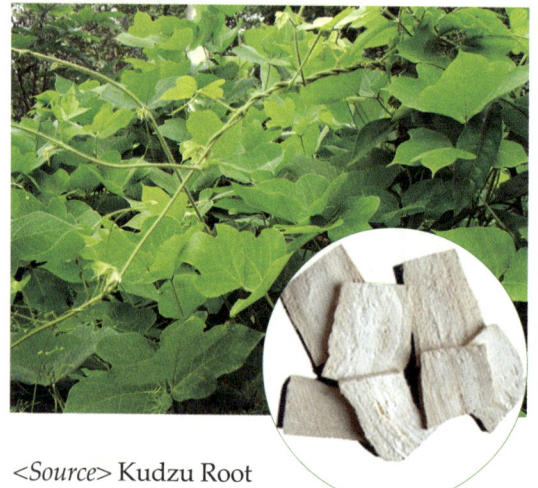

<Source> Kudzu Root

<Property> sweet, acrid, cool

Kudzu root is now a common plant in many parts of the world and is even considered a serious problem in the American south due to its unstoppable growth. It can be used in cooking, as medicine, and even as animal feed! Medicinally it is commonly used in treating the common cold, but in diabetes it is useful because it can relieve thirst without harming the digestive system. It is listed among the 50 most important medicinals in Chinese medicine.

<Pharmacology studies>

Flavones extracted from *gě gēn* can increase blood flow to cerebral and coronary vessels and reduce resistance so as to lower blood pressure. Another component, daidzein, can persistently reduce blood sugar levels in diabetic mice.

Huáng lián (Rhizoma Coptidis)

<Source> Coptis Rhizome

<Property> bitter, cold

Known as one of the bitterest substances in the Chinese repitiore, the taste of *huáng lián* may take some getting used to. But its ability to clear heat from the body is unrivaled which makes it very useful in the treatment of diabetes. It can both quench the thirst and relieve the hunger that diabetic patients suffer from. *Huáng lián* is also often used in the treatment of bacterial infections which usually present as heat in the body.

<Pharmacology studies>

Huáng lián's major component, berberine, can lower blood sugar levels significantly in normal and diabetic mice. Experiments show that berberine takes effect through inhibiting glyconeogenesis and promoting glucolysis rather than affecting insulin secretion or its receptor performance.

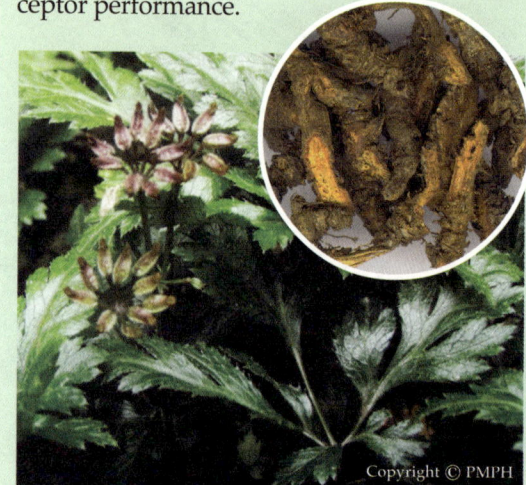

Sāng bái pí (Cortex Mori)

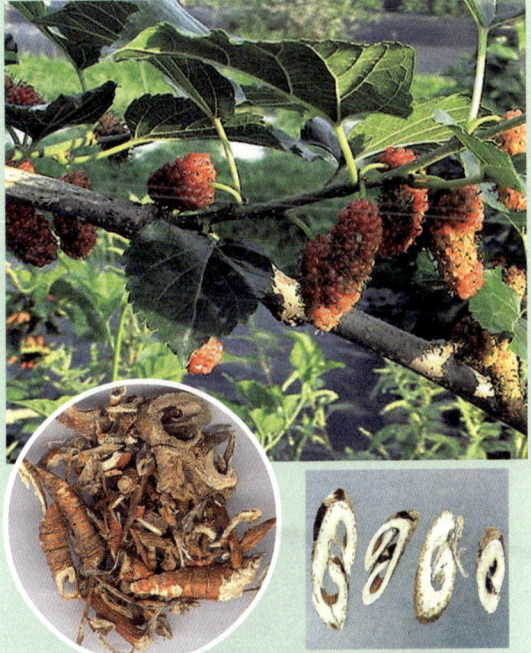

<Source> Mulberry Tree Root Bark

<Property> sweet, cold

The famous Mulberry tree, whose leaves are the food of silkworms, is the source of numerous medicinals. The root bark specifically is used to clear heat from the upper body. This function, plus information gained from recent research, makes it useful in the treatment of diabetes.

<Pharmacology studies>

Sāng bái pí has the effect of lowering blood sugar levels according to a research on 50 anti-diabetic herbs by Beijing Hospital.

Tiān huā fěn (Radix Trichosanthis)

<Source> Snakegourd Root

<Property> bitter, slightly sweet, cold

"The powder of heavenly flowers" is this herb's poetic name in Chinese. While not one of the main substances used in diabetes, it makes a great addition to any formula if a patient has excessive thirst. With such a wonderful name, anyone would welcome it in their decoction.

<Pharmacology studies>

When used alone, *tiān huā fěn* is not effective in reducing blood sugar levels. When paired with other herbs, it can be effective.

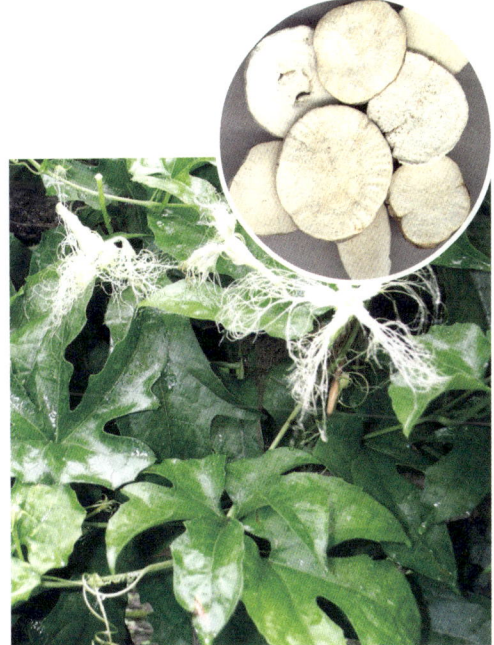

2. What Will My Treatment Program Be Like?

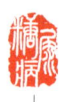

Chinese medicinals are the mainstay of Chinese medicine. Although acupuncture is the best known modality here in the West, in China the great majority of patients who seek treatment from Chinese medicine get herbal formulas. Treatment with herbal medicine is thought to have a wider scope than the more commonly known acupuncture, and for most diseases it works faster. Another, more practical advantage of treatment with Chinese medicinals is the frequency of office visits. Acupuncture patients are frequently seen two or three times per week, while herbal prescriptions are usually modified once a week, with visits becoming even less frequent as the patient's condition stabilizes.

Similar to the modalities that work on the points and channels like acupuncture, moxibustion, cupping, etc, herbal medicine can be administered in many different ways. The most common method is done by taking the raw herbs, boiling them to extract their effective properties, and then drinking the resulting liquid. Chinese medicine calls this a "decoction". In general, taking Chinese medicinals as a decoction is the most potent and fastest working form of treatment available.

Since treatment methods vary greatly from disease to disease, and styles differ between practitioners, the exact amounts of herbs, number of packets, and preparation instructions will likewise be very different. Here we are trying to give a general idea about a typical treatment. If your practitioner gives you something that falls outside the guidelines listed here, do not be concerned.

Preparation of the decoction

At the practitioner's office, you will most likely be given several packets of Chinese medicinals. Each packet will be for 1-2 days use and will probably contain from 70-120 grams of herbs. Take the time to examine the herbs in the packet. Enjoy the different colors, smells, and textures. As many Chinese medicinals are common plants found around the world, you may even find something you recognize. Being able to get to know your medicine and the ability to be involved in its preparation is one thing that never fails to endear a patient to Chinese medicine.

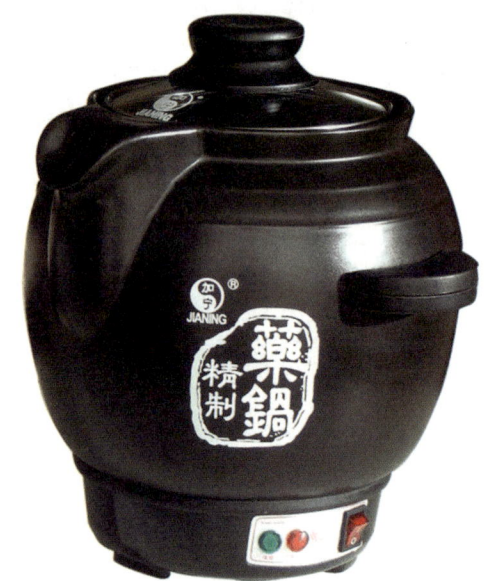

Electrical Decoction Pot

To cook the decoction, first put all the medicinals into a ceramic or glass pot (metal is not suitable) and add water until it completely covers the medicinals (your practitioner may tell you an exact amount of water to add). The mixture should be brought to a boil on high heat and then reduced to a medium flame. Usually the decoction needs to be boiled for 20-60 minutes depending on the ingredients of the formula. Strain the decoction, divide the liquid in two, and drink it twice a day in two equal portions, usually once before breakfast and once after dinner. Most often, one packet is one day's dosage. Sometimes you will be asked to save the dregs to be cooked again in the future. In this case, they should be stored in the refrigerator.

There are some ingredients that have special cooking instructions such as cooking alone for 20-30 minutes before other ingredients are added (for especially dense materials), those that should be added at the last five minutes of cooking (for very delicate medicinals), or those that should be added last to the strained decoction (for materials in powder, gel, or liquid form).

Medicinals have long been prepared in this way for thousands of years in China. It is not a simple mixture of herbs. During cooking, complex chemical reactions are happening. Effective ingredients are released from the herbs. Components may also act on each other. It is still not possible to get the exact picture of the whole process. Yet clinical experience have proven that they are safe and effective.

Recently, some clinics offer a decoction cooking service. The decoction will be made by a machine and sealed in plastic bags to store in the refrigerator.

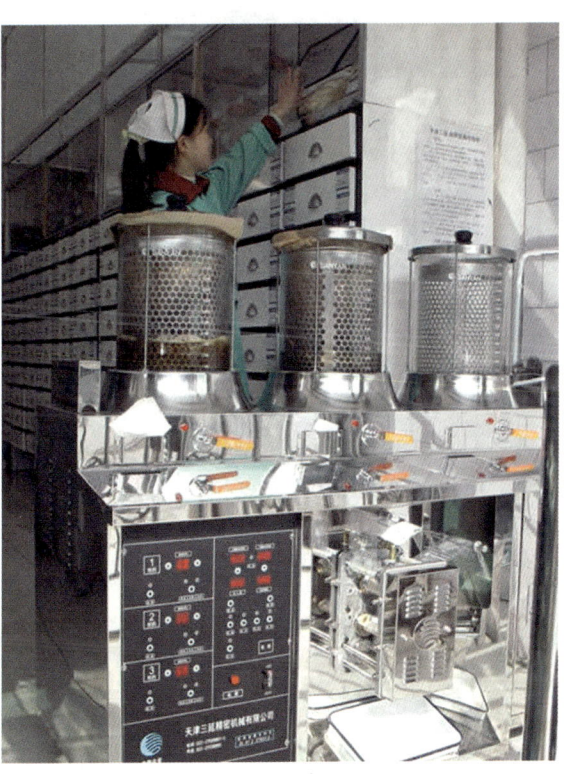

Decoction Machines

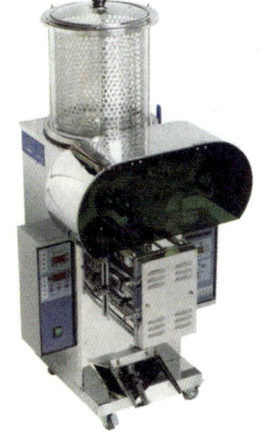
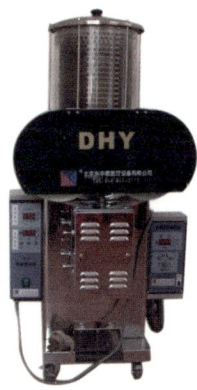

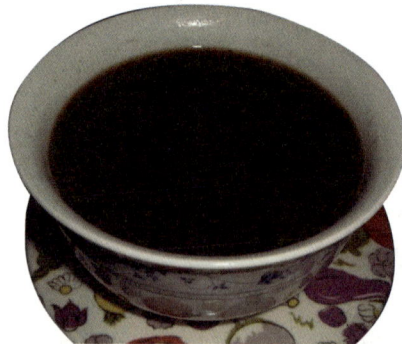

No matter if you or the clinic prepares the herbs, when you drink your decoction it should be warm. Only in special cases is room temperature acceptable.

Treatment course

For chronic diseases, decoctions take time to have an effect. When you go to the clinic for the first time, the practitioner will usually give a prescription for 3-7 days. Each day's dose should be divided into two equal parts, usually taken in the morning and evening. You will need to come back to the clinic about once a week for the practitioner to modify the prescription. After a month or so has passed, you and your practitioner will reevaluate your condition and your treatment strategy may change allowing for gradually smaller amounts of medicinals, and more infrequent office visits. A treatment course usually lasts a few months, but may be more or less depending on the severity of the case.

You are advised to take the decoction about 1 hour before meals. If the decoction irritates your stomach, take it after meals. The timing may vary with the specific prescription, but generally speaking, it is common to take the decoction once in the morning before breakfast and once at night before going to bed. Warm up the liquid before you drink it.

At first you may find the making of your decoction troublesome, and/or have a strong dislike of the unfamiliar taste. This is a common problem, especially in the west where we are accustomed to our medicine being easy to take and either tasteless or sugar coated. We can only ask that you recall the millions of people who have benefited from this treatment method and give a fair trial, at least two weeks, to the decoction method. In fact, it is the experience of many doctors and patients that if the prescription properly fits the imbalance, the initially unfamiliar or unpleasant taste will become something the patient enjoys and looks forward to.

Formulas for the most commonly seen patterns in diabetes mellitus

A typical formula consists of between 5 to 15 ingredients with each ingredient usually dosed between 6 and 30 grams. The ingredients in the formula are arranged according to a hierarchy. The chief ingredient represents the main therapeutic effect and will often have the largest dose. The assistants and deputies either support the chief, address another aspect of the imbalance, or perform a checking action against some other ingredient that may be too harsh in some way. The last soldier, the courier, serves to guide the formula to a certain body part, organ, or channel, or acts to harmonize the formula. See if you can recognize some of the single herbs mentioned above in the formulas below.

Deficiency of yin fluids

<Typical manifestations>: strong thirst, dry mouth, dry stool, dark yellow urine, a red tongue with little coating, and a fine rapid pulse.

Table 4-2 *Zēng Yè Tāng* (Increase Fluids Decoction)

Medicinal	Pinyin	Dose	Latin Name
Figwort Root	xuán shēn	30g	Radix Scrophulariae
Dwarf Lilyturf Tuber	mài dōng	24g	Radix Ophiopogonis
Raw Rehmannia Root	shēng dì huáng	24g	Radix Rehmanniae

This formula is aimed to increase yin fluids. *Mài dōng* and *shēng dì huáng* serve to purpose. *Xuán shēn* is used to clear heat to better supplement yin.

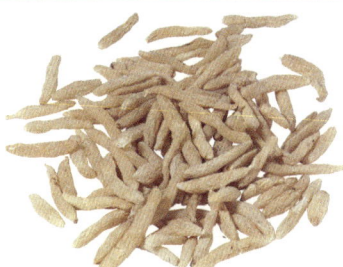
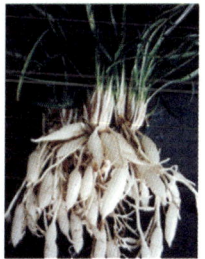

mài dōng (Dwarf Lilyturf Tuber)

Extreme heat due to yin deficiency

<*Typical manifestations*>: severe thirst, bitter taste in the mouth, agitation and irritability, constipation, dark yellow urine, a red tongue with little coating, and a fine rapid pulse

Table 4-3 *Modified Bái Hǔ Tāng* (White Tiger Decoction)

Medicinal	Pinyin	Dose	Latin Name
Gypsum	shí gāo	30g	Gypsum Fibrosum
Common Anemarrhena Rhizome	zhī mǔ	9g	Rhizoma Anemarrhenae
Liquorice Root	gān cǎo	3g	Radixet Rhizoma Glycyrrhizae
Rice	Jīng mǐ	9g	Rice
Baical Skullcap Root	huáng qín	10g	Radix Scutellariae
Chinese Wolfberry Root-Bark	dì gǔ pí	10g	Cortex Lycii
Radix Ophiopogonis	mài mén dōng	15g	Radix Ophiopogonis
Trichosanthin	tiān huā fěn	15g	Radix Trichosanthis

The basis of this formula was created nearly 2000 years ago by arguably the most famous Chinese doctor of all time. Originally it was made to treat high fevers, but with some modification it treats diabetes where the heat is severe and the yin is deficient. In addition to two medicinals discussed above (*dì gǔ pí, tiān huā fěn*), this formula contains licorice root whose sweet nature is used to harmonize a formula's ingredients.

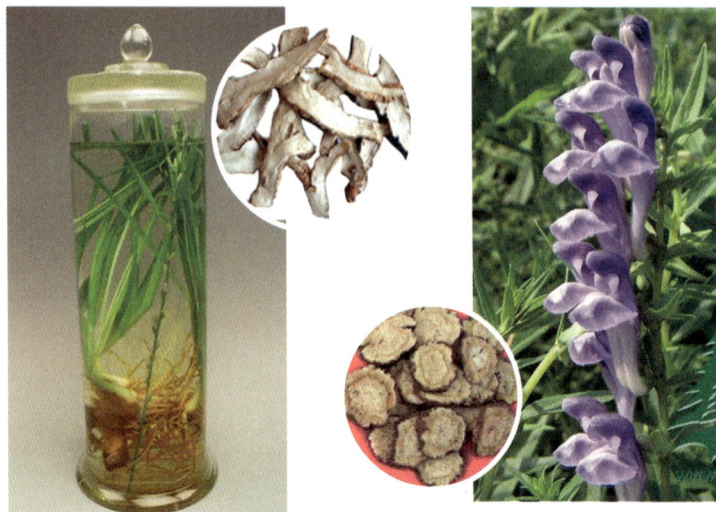

zhī mǔ (Common Anemarrhena Rhizome)   *huáng qín* (Baical Skullcap Root)

Deficiency of qi and yin

<*Typical manifestations*>: fatigue, weakness, lassitude, excessive sweating on slight exertion, abdominal distension, loose stool, a pale tongue and whitish coating, in addition to other manifestations of yin deficiency as mentioned above.

Table 4-4 *Shēng Mài Sǎn* (Powder to Give Life to the Pulse)

Medicinal	*Pinyin*	Dose	Latin Name
Ginseng	*rén shēn*	10g	Radix et Rhizoma Ginseng
Tuber of Dwarf Lilyturf	*mài dōng*	15g	Radix Ophiopogonis
Chinese Magnolivine Fruit	*wǔ wèi zǐ*	6g	Fructus Schisandrae Chinensis

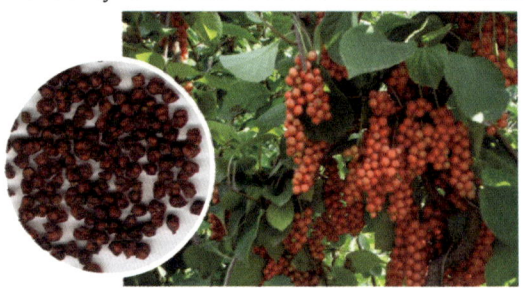

wǔ wèi zǐ (Chinese Magnolivine Fruit)

A model of elegant formula construction, *Shēng Mài Sǎn* has one ingredient to strengthen qi, one to nourish yin, and one to make sure qi and yin stay properly in the body. In moderate doses, this formula is used for those who have weak qi and yin; but in higher doses it is used in emergency medicine to do exactly what its name says it does, give life to the pulse. In China it is even given in IV form.

Deficiency of qi and yin with stagnation

<Typical manifestations>: the above symptoms of qi and yin deficiency plus symptoms of blocked channels and collaterals such as numbness and pain of the limbs, or atrophy of the muscles.

This is an example (Table 4-5) of a formula that was specially made to treat diabetes patients. It addresses the main patterns seen in diabetes (qi and yin deficiency plus blood stagnation) and makes use of medicinals that are known to lower blood sugar levels. This is modern Chinese medicine at its finest.

Deficiency of yin and yang

<Typical Manifestation>: Fatigue, weakness, soreness in the lower back and knees, a hot sensation in the palms and soles, a cold sensation on the back of the palms and soles, a pale tongue, and a deep fine pulse.

To treat this serious condition, two formulas are used and both can be taken in pill form. The first is a prescription put together by a famous (Table 4-6) physician from the Tang dynasty (roughly 1400 years ago) who is still known as the "Herbal King". This formula treats a weakened kidney's yin and yang aspects simultaneously. The second formula is a simple combination that prevents the leakage of fluids that would further weaken the body.

Table 4-5 *Yì Qì Yǎng Yīn Huó Xuè Tāng*
(Boost Qi Nourish Yin Move Blood Decoction)

Medicinal	Pinyin	Dose	Latin Name
Solomonsela Rhizome	huáng jīng	3g	Rhizoma Polygonati
Milkvetch Root	huáng qí	30g	Radix Astragali
Heterophylly Falsesatarwort Root	tài zǐ shēn	15g	Radix Pseudostellariae
Dwarf Lilyturf Tuber	mài dōng	12g	Radix Ophiopogonis
Chinese Magnolivine Fruit	wǔ wèi zǐ	10g	Fructus Schisandrae Sphenantherae
Rehmannia Dride Rhizome	shēng dì huáng	20g	Radix Rehmanniac Recens
Figwort Root	xuán shēn	30g	Radix Scrophulariae
Danshen Root	dān shēn	30g	Radix et Rhizoma Salviae Miltiorrhizae
Chinese Angelica	dāng guī	10g	Radix Angelicae Sinensis
Peach Seed	táo rén	10g	Semen Persicae
Kudzuvine Root	gě gēn	15g	Radix Puerariae Lobatae
Trichosanthin	tiān huā fěn	30g	Radix Trichosanthis
Immature Orange Fruit	zhǐ shí	10g	Fructus Aurantii Immaturus
Raw Rhubarb	dà huáng	6g	Radix et Rhizoma Rhei

Table 4-6 *Jīn Kuì Shèn Qì Wán* with *Shuǐ Lù Èr Xiān Dān*
(Land and Sea Two Immortals Pills)

Medicinal	Pinyin	Dose	Latin name
Rehmannia Dried Root	dì huáng	240g	Radix Rehmanniae
Chinese Yam	shān yào	120g	Rhizoma Dioscoreae
Asiatic Cornlian Cherry Fruit	shān zhū yú	120g	Fructus Corni
Oriental Waterplantain Rhizome	zé xiè	90g	Rhizoma Alismatis
Indian Bread	fú líng	90g	Poria
Tree Peony Bark	mǔ dān pí	90g	Cortex Moutan
Cassia Twig	guì zhī	30g	Cinnamomi
Prepared Common Monkshood Daughter Root	fù zǐ (prepared)	30g	Radix Aconiti Praeparata
Gordon Euryale seed	qiàn shí	30g	Semen Euryales
Cherokee Rose Fruit	yīng zǐ	30g	Fructus Rosae laevigatae

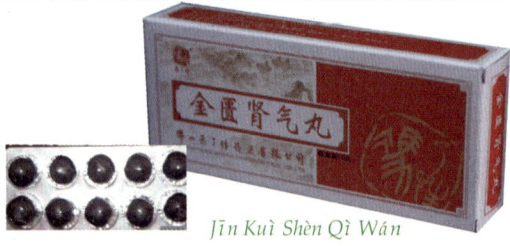

Jīn Kuì Shèn Qì Wán

Other forms of Chinese medicinals -Prepared medicines

Prepared medicines usually come in the form of pills or tablets, though some are given as syrups or powders. This is probably the easiest way to take Chinese medicinals as it is similar to taking a western pharmaceutical. The practitioner gives you the bottle (or bottles) of pills, tells you how many to take and how often, and when the time comes, you simply take the proper number of pills with warm water. The advantages over decoctions are obvious as you can avoid the cooking process and the strange taste. The major disadvantage may not be as obvious, but it is significant.

The reason Chinese medicine is so effective is that treatment can be tailored to exactly match the patient's individual pattern of disharmony. With Chinese medicinals, this is achieved by blending together a combination of substances that correspond to the presenting patterns. While formulas are helpful in that they serve as a guide to the treatment of the most common patterns, in almost all cases a formula will need to be modified to fit the patient exactly. The formula represented in a bottle of prepared medicine is unlikely to perfectly line up with a given patient's condition. Some parts of the patient's condition may remain unaddressed, and some parts of the formula may be inappropriate for the patient. This is why prepared medicines are usually used near the end of treatment, in order to "consolidate the treatment effect" by giving mild, long-term treatment directed at the patient's primary pattern. That being said, some practitioners combine two, three, or even more different prepared medicines to more accurately cover the patient's presentation.

Take, as an example, a patient with qi and yin deficiency who also has qi stagnation and heat in the liver channel. The practitioner may choose to use the formula *Shēng Mài Sǎn* that was described above as the base formula to strengthen qi and yin and modify it to also remove stagnation and clear heat, given as a decoction. After a few months, when the patient's condition is brought under control, the practitioner might decide to have the patient take a small daily dose of the prepared version of *Shēng Mài Sǎn* to taper off the treatment by continuing to concentrate on the main patterns.

Another patient, this one also with qi and yin deficiency, but in this case the yin deficiency and dryness are severe. If the patient is unable to cook decoctions, the practitioner may decide to give the patient two different prepared medicines. *Shēng Mài Sǎn* could be given to treat the qi and yin deficiency, and *Zēng Yè Tāng* may be given as well to concentrate on the extreme dryness, both in pill form.

There are a total of 13 antidiabetic prepared medicines of plant origin that have been officially approved by the Chinese FDA for commercial use in China. See Table 4-7.

Table 4-7 Prepared Medicines

English Name
Shen qi jiang tang powder
Jiang tang jia tablet
Jiang tang shu capsule
Jin qi jiang tang tablet
Ke le ning capsule
Tang mai kang powder
Xiao ke an capsule
Xiao ke ping tablet
Xiao ke wan
Xiao tang ling capsule
Yang yin jiang tang tablet
Yu quan wan
Qi zhi jiang tang capsule

These formulas contain many different combinations of medicinals, but since they are all designed specifically for diabetes patients, they have much in common. Since the most common presentation of patterns in a diabetes patient is yin deficiency with qi deficiency, every one of these products contains medicinals that strengthen the body's yin and qi. Also, since internal heat, stagnation, and kidney weakness are also common, many of these patterns are addressed. Since each product is slightly different, a trained professional will need to help you choose the best one.

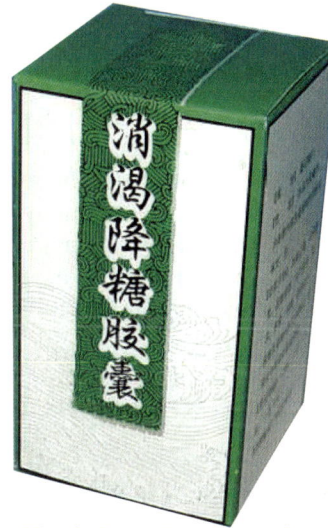

Xiao ke Jiang Tang capsule

Granules

Chinese medicinals in granule form is a modern creation and represents a middle path between decoctions and prepared medicines. To make granules, individual herbs or whole formulas are cooked down until a concentrated powder remains. These are packaged and can be combined to fit the patient's exact pattern. The patient takes the granule packets, empties them into a cup or container, pours hot water over the mixture, stirs to dissolve, and drinks. This allows a more convenient preparation, and individualized formula design. However, it is generally thought that taking herbs in granule form is slightly less effective than decoctions. Despite this, granules have become popular with many patients and practitioners in recent years due to their ease of preparation.

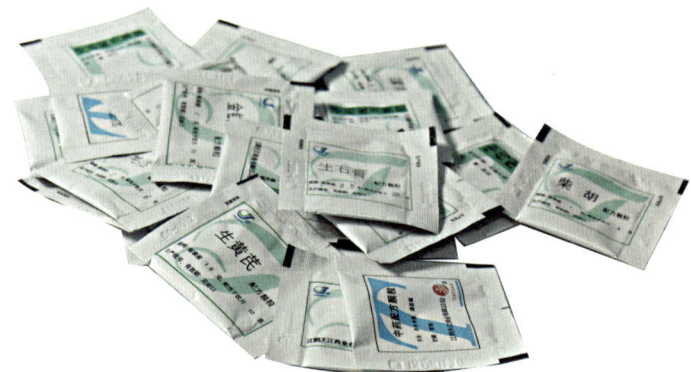

External Application

Chinese medicinals are sometimes prepared so that they may be applied directly to the skin to be absorbed superficially. External applications are usually used for problems of the skin and superficial channels. They are used often in dermatology, but are also often used to treat pain, numbness, and injury of a local area. Patients with diabetes may be given a formula to use externally in order to treat neuropathy.

The simplest way to make an external application is to boil herbs like you would a decoction and apply the cooled liquid to the skin. This can then be wrapped in gauze for a better effect. External applications do not need to be as specific as decoctions that are taken internally. For this reason, many practitioners use some kind of prepared medicine, usually prepared as an alcohol extract, an oil, a cream, or sometimes as a plaster that will stick to the body. Foot soaks using Chinese medicinal formulas have proven to be very effective in treating diabetic neuropathy.

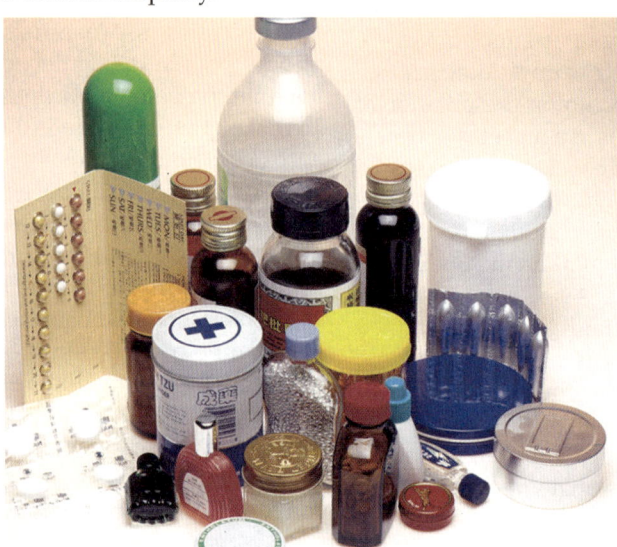

Attention
The information in this section is not meant to be a cookbook for you to choose from. It is presented in order to help you understand more about Chinese medicine. The selection of medicinals must be done by a trained Chinese medical practitioner.

3. Translated Research

(1) A study in Tianjin, China, in 2006 among a group of 62 patients with diabetes mellitus showed that by using Chinese herbal medicine along with dietary restriction over a course of 6 months, their blood sugar was lowered by an average of 0.46 mmol/L (8.3 mg/dl) over a control group that received only dietary restriction.

(2) A study in Hubei, China, in 2004 among a group of 160 patients with diabetes showed that by using Chinese medicinal treatment based on pattern identification compared with biomedical treatment (Gilemal and Metformin) over a course of 3 months, 88.6% of this group had some improvement over a control group with a 50.9% effective rate that received only biomedicine (effective: fasting plasma glucose dropped below 8.3mmol/L) (149.4 mg/dl), 2h plasma glucose 10 mmol/L (180mg/dl), or blood sugar dropped more than 10%).

(3) A study in Xinjiang, China, in 2003 among a group of 62 patients with diabetes mellitus showed that by using Chinese herbal medicine for only 2 months, their blood sugar was lowered by an average of 0.53 mmol/L (9.5 mg/dl) over a control group that received only biomedicine. No significant difference was found between using western medicine and using Chinese medicinals.

(4) A study in Nanjing, China, in 1995 among a group of 90 patients with diabetes showed that by using Chinese medicinals along with biomedical treatment over a course of 1 month their blood sugar lowered by an average of 0.56 mmol/L (10.1 mg/dl) over a control group that received only biomedicine.

(5) A study in Nanjing, China, in 2003 among a group of 60 patients with diabetes mellitus showed that by using Chinese herbal medicine solely over a course of 1 month, their blood sugar was lowered by an average of 0.49 mmol/L (8.8 mg/dl) over a control group that received only biomedicine. No significant difference was found between using biomedicine and using Chinese medicinals.

(6) A study in Guangdong, China, in 2002 among a group of 405 patients with diabetes showed that by using Chinese herbal medicine solely over a course of 1 month, their blood sugar was lowered by an average of 2.58 mmol/L (46.4 mg/dl) over a control group that received only biomedicine. The efficacy of Chinese medicine as compared to biomedical treatment of diabetes mellitus showed no significant difference.

(7) A study in Henan, China, between 2001 and 2004 among a group of 80 patients with diabetes showed that by using Chinese herbal medicine along with biomedical treatment over a course of 2 months, their blood sugar was lowered by an average of 2.2 mmol/L (39.6 mg/dl) over a control group that received only biomedicine.

(8) A study in Sichuan,

China, in 2004 studied a group of 60 patients with diabetes and 30 healthy volunteers. The results showed that by using Chinese herbal medicine along with biomedical treatment over a course of 1 month, their blood sugar was lowered by an average of 6.48 mmol/L (116.64 mg/dl) over a control group of diabetic patients that received only biomedicine.

(9) A study in Shanxi, China, in 2001 among a group of 56 patients with diabetes mellitus showed that by using Chinese herbal medicine along with biomedical treatment over a course of 3 months, blood and urine sugar levels could be returned to normal. The total effective rate was 94.6%. It showed that the use of Chinese herbal medicine had strengthened the efficacy of the biomedical drugs.

(10) A study in Hunan, China, between 2004 and 2007 among a group of 60 patients with diabetes showed that by using Chinese herbal medicine along with biomedical treatment over a course of 1 month, their blood sugar was lowered by an average of 4.77 mmol/L (85.86 mg/dl) over a control group that received only biomedicine.

(11) A study in Shanghai, China, in 2000 among a group of 70 patients with diabetes showed that by using Chinese herbal medicine along with biomedical treatment over a course of 3 months, their fasting serum glucose was lowered by an average of 3.64 mmol/L (65.52 mg/dl) over a control group that received only biomedicine.

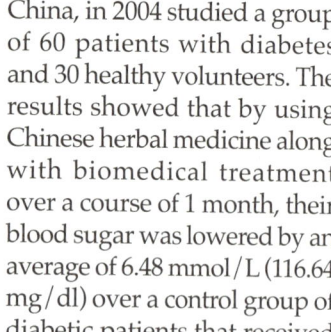

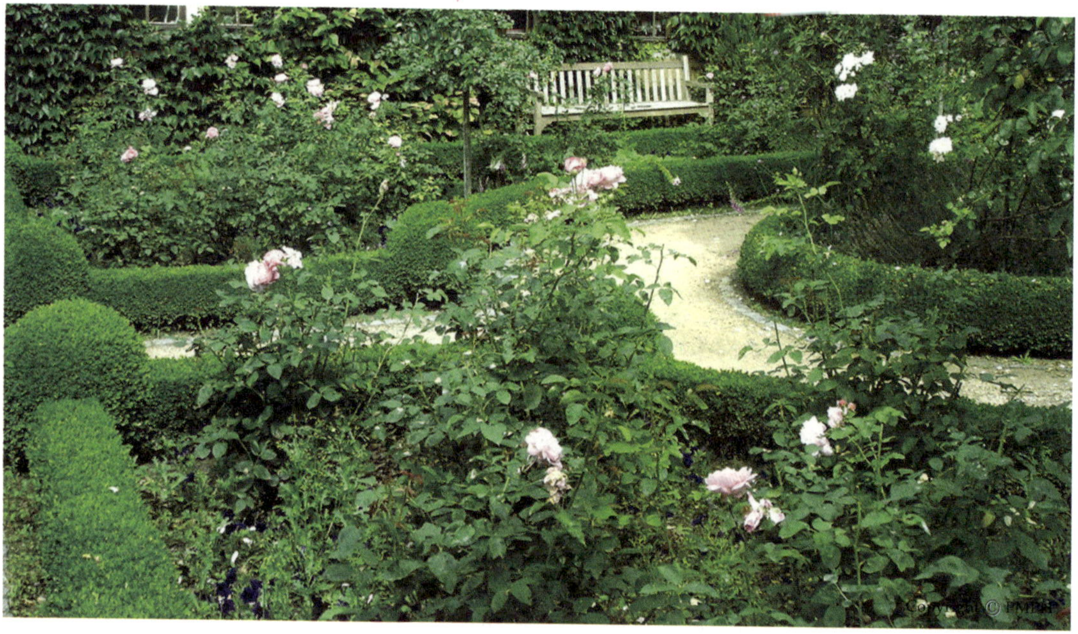

Tui Na (Massage)

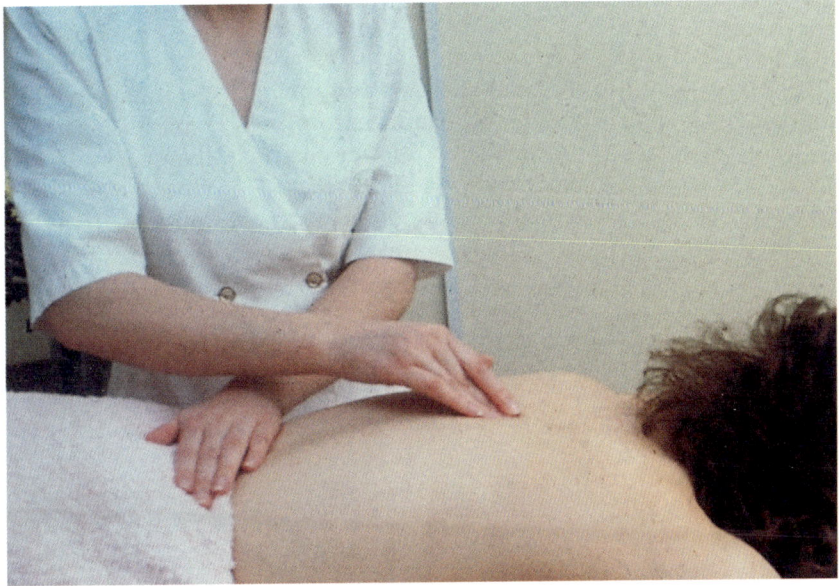

Tui na, literally "pushing and grasping", but better translated as massage, is a manual practice of manipulating the body performed by highly-skilled practitioners. By stimulating the specific areas (acupuncture points or channels) with well-honed techniques, the channels can be opened and the flow of qi and blood will be promoted and regulated. The body's qi will be strengthened and so will its resistance to disease. Tui na is an important element of Chinese medicine and is popular with everyday people as it is simple, convenient, effective, and cheap.

Tui na is irreplaceable as a natural kind of physical therapy. You may have already tried other kinds of massage, but the tui na of Chinese medicine is unique because it is deeply rooted in Chinese medical theory. For example, according to the theory of Chinese medicine, pain is either due to stagnation or deficiency, and local stagnation of the flow of qi and blood is the most common cause. Tui na can relieve this kind of pain by applying forceful, regular, smooth, and penetrating manipulations in order to remove stagnation and promote the flow of qi and blood. Pain with a different diagnosis would be treated differently, in accordance to theory. As in all aspects of Chinese medicine, applying individualized treatment is of primary importance. Discovering the unique pattern of disharmony in each patient is vital in order to apply the correct treatment methods.

In the treatment of diabetes, tui na is effective, though it often plays a supplementary role. Manual stimulus on the acupuncture points (acupressure) will also produce effects similar to acupuncture according to the theory of Chinese medicine. Tui na is more convenient and also may sound safer if you are afraid of needles. What's more important is it is at least as effective as needles. A survey in India among 493 diabetic patients revealed that among the nearly 70% who had tried complementary or alternative therapies, acupressure was felt to have been the most beneficial. Small scale studies done in mainland China have shown that tui na can greatly relieve the symptoms of diabetes and even reduce the dosage of biomedical medication. If applied regularly, tui na can not only relieve your symptoms, but can contribute to the management of blood sugar levels. It will make you feel comfortable, relaxed and refreshed every time you leave the clinic. You will know how well tui na works once you try it.

1. What Will My Treatment Program Be Like?

After inquiring about your condition and performing a detailed examination, the practitioner will decide on a tui na procedure based on the pattern identification. Since tui na is a direct, manual therapy, treatment can take place almost anywhere and in many positions, but most often the patients will be asked to lie on their back or stomach. Sometimes the massage will be done in the sitting position. If necessary, the position may be changed during the treatment.

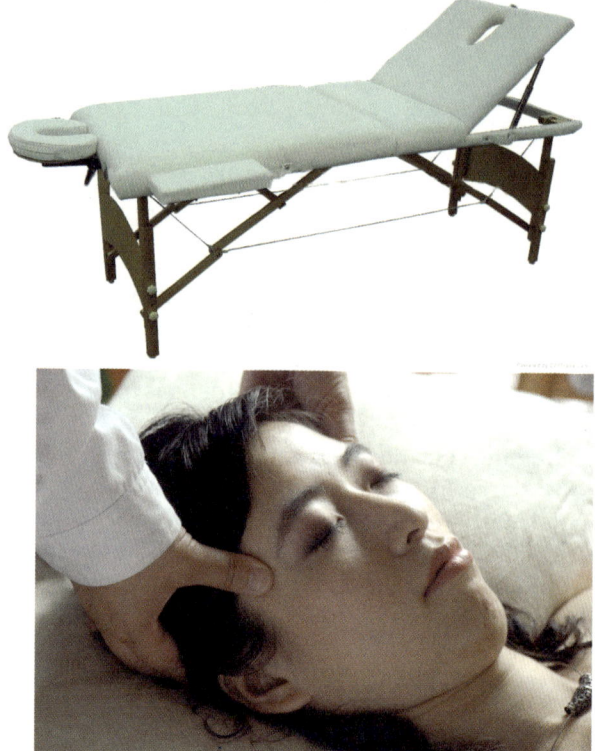

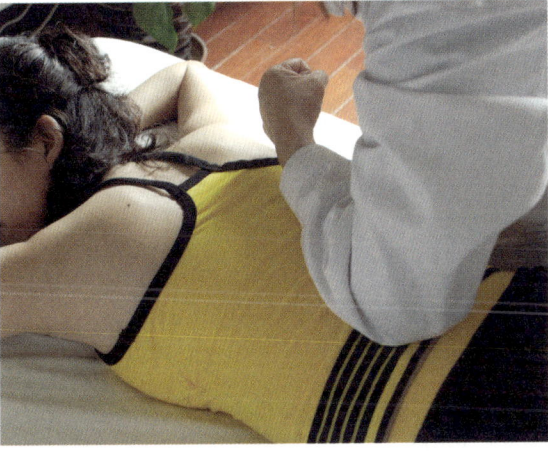
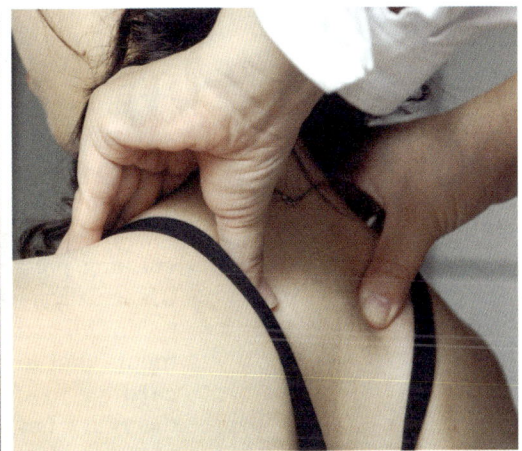

A pair of trained hands is all that is necessary for a tui na treatment to be performed. That's why the manipulations are called "*shou fa*" (techniques of the hands) in Chinese. Other parts of the practitioner's body might also be used, such as elbows and arms. Occasionally, a practitioner might use some kind of massage tools.

Special oil or medicinal paste may sometimes be used to lubricate and protect the skin and for their own therapeutic effects. The most common ingredients are common oily substances like lanolin or beeswax mixed with herbs that invigorate qi and blood. If you are allergic to certain substances, please inform the practitioner before treatment begins. Sometimes medicinal pastes are specially made to treat certain conditions. For example, one kind of paste for deficiency pain, another for stagnation pain; one kind for the upper body and a different type for the lower half.

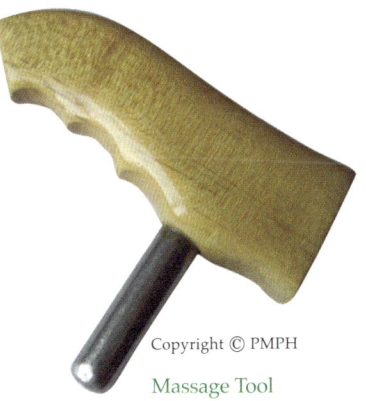
Massage Tool

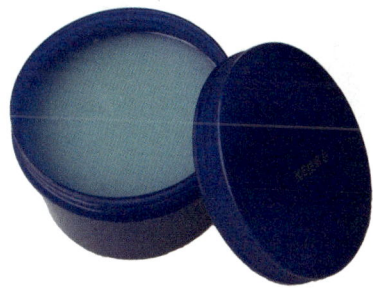
Massage Cream

2. At Home Massage

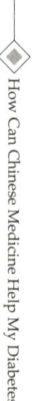

Techniques of manipulation and point selection will be made on the basis of the patient's condition and existing patterns. Since the fundamental pathomachnism of diabetes in Chinese medicine is yin deficiency, points and techniques that can supplement yin will usually be part of the treatment. Other points will be chosen according to the patient's pattern diagnosis or symptoms.

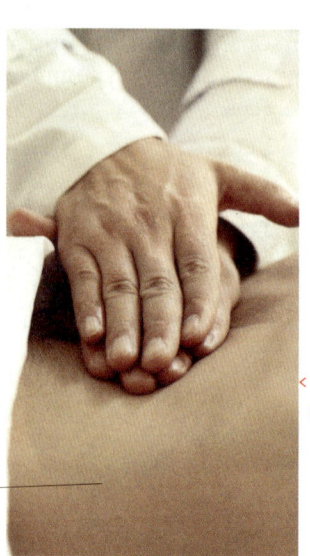

Tui na manipulation is not as simple as it looks, even though many of the procedures look similar to actions performed every day such as pushing, grasping, pressing and kneading. It is actually a set of highly-skilled techniques and expert movements that are performed according to Chinese medical theory. It is targeted at the system of channels and acupuncture points throughout the body. Therefore, the manipulation must be performed by trained practitioners to promote internal self-adjustment of the channel system without harming the local tissues of the body.

The effect of tui na depends more on the skill with which the manipulations are performed rather on the sheer force of the pressure. Force, even a small amount, applied improperly can be harmful to the body. It is possible to see patients, who have been treated by "tui na therapy" offered by non-professional practitioners, with bruises or other accidents. It is not suggested to perform or receive tui na treatments that you have observed in the clinic on or by your friends or family members without the presence of an instructor.

Nonetheless, there are some self-massage practices which are safe, simple, convenient, and designed for diabetic patients to exercise their body and mind, regulate organ function, and serve as a supplement to the management of diabetes.

There are many different manipulations in tui na, and hundreds of acupuncture points and body parts these techniques can be used on. To make things simple, we have chosen one protocol that can be performed on the patient by a friend or family member, and one routine that can be performed by the patient themselves. Please note that there are numerous tui na routines and self-massage protocols recommended for diabetic patients. We have tried to choose two that have some evidence of their effectiveness, but routines learned from your practitioner or other sources may work as well. The most important thing is to find something that helps you and feels good.

The first protocol was used in a study on diabetes that was reported to be effective. The study employed the following procedure every other day for 30 minutes each time.

(1) Use the rolling method on the bladder channel (running parallel to the spine on both sides) on the back for 10 minutes. To perform this method, use a loose fist and roll up and down the back. This area is home to an important group of points that connect to each internal organ. Massage of this area can help to harmonize the entire body.

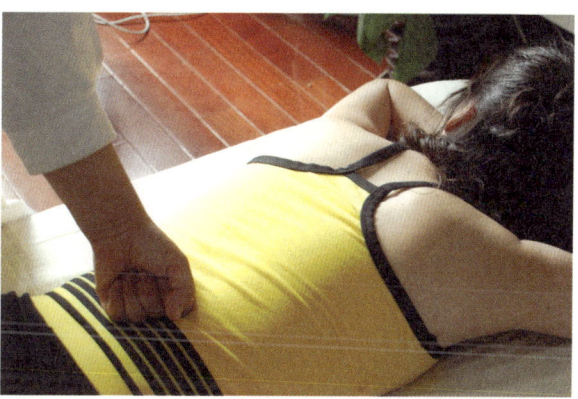

(2) First locate tender areas of the back by pressing. Then flick and pluck these points. Lastly, rub laterally on the kidney point *shèn shù* (BL 23) which lies about two fingers out from the spine roughly level to the belly button on the back. The kidney is a very important organ, especially for diabetics. Working on this point will help to strengthen this precious organ. Other tender points are where the qi and blood has become stuck. Chronic stagnation can affect the internal organs. Better to relieve that stagnation now!

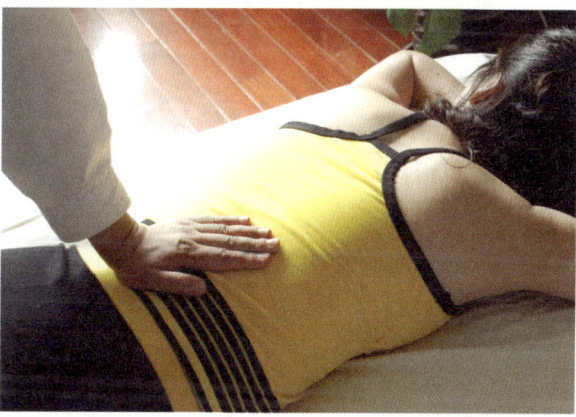

(3) Rub in a circular motion on the abdomen for 15 minutes. The abdomen is home to many important organs of digestion that are central to healthy qi. Rubbing this area gently will help to strengthen the body's qi.

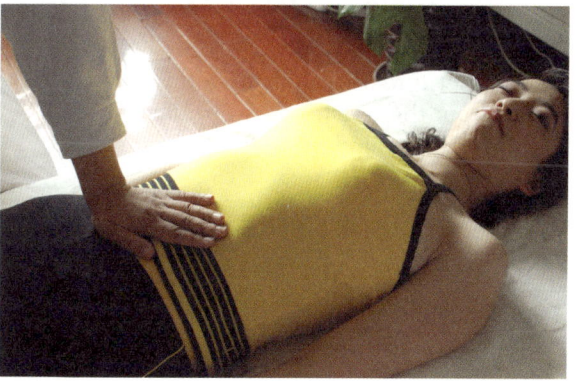

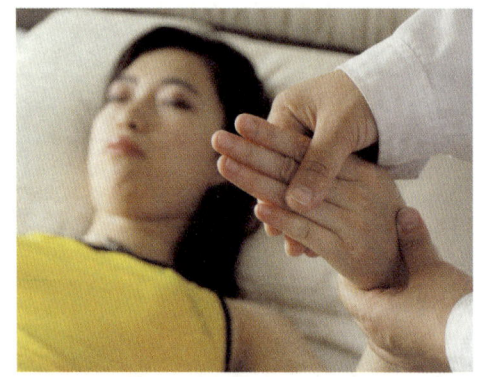
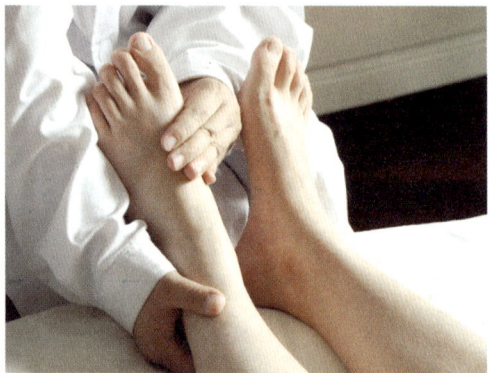

(4) Perform acupressure on the reflex point of the pancreas on the feet and hands for 2 minutes. Please see the pictures for the location of the pancreas reflex point on the feet and hands.

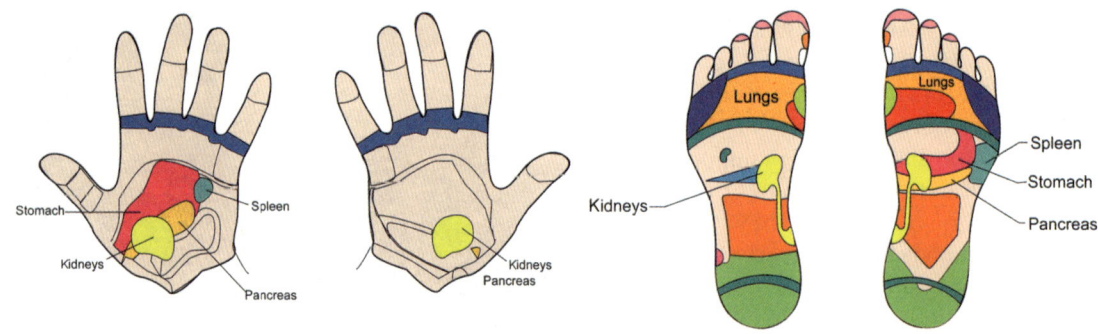

(5) Flick and pluck the point *nèi guān* **(PC 6) 12 times.** *Nèi guān* (PC 6) is located on the inner forearm, about two finger-widths from the wrist, and is primarily used to relax the mind and calm the heart.

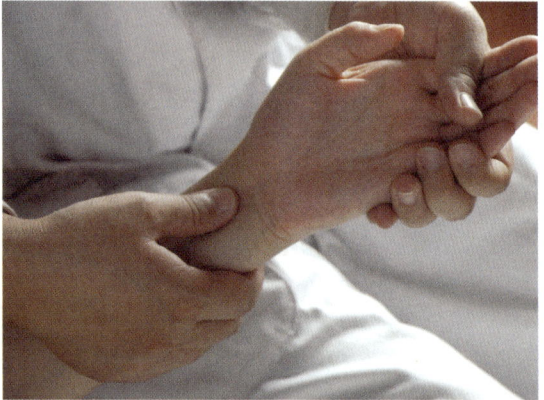

This procedure should take about 30 minutes per session.

Self Massage

This self-massage protocol is recommended by a Chinese text on the treatment of diabetes.

(1) Pre-massage

Stand with the feet roughly shoulder width apart. Relax the whole body and calm down the mind. Relax the muscles of the face. Touch the upper palate (the place inside the mouth where the gums meet the teeth) with your tongue. Look straight ahead. Close the eyes gently and stay still for 3 minutes.

Sit down to practice this exercise when you are not feeling well or at an advanced stage of diabetes.

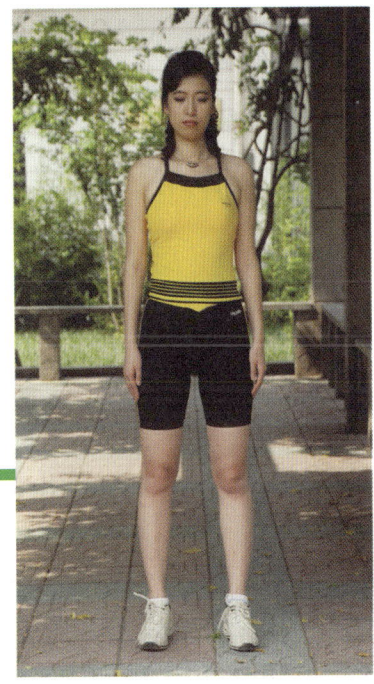

(2) Massage

1) *Dān tián* breathing

Put both of your palms over the *dān tián*. Take 3 deep, long, gentle, even breaths. During each breathing, guide your breath deep down to the *dān tián* area with your mind. Then extend both hands outward and then back to cover the *dān tián* again. Do this three times. This is to regulate your breath.

Dān tián is usually translated as "Elixir Field" but literally means "Cinnabar Field". This area, important to all forms of Asian healing, exercise, and martial arts, is located inside the abdomen roughly three inches (10cm) below the navel. This is where the root of health exists and can be nourished.

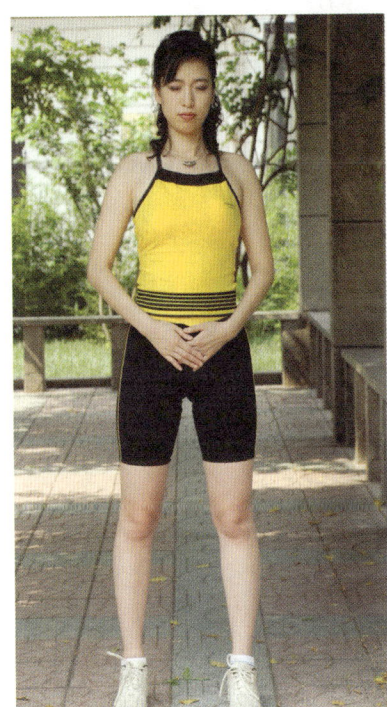

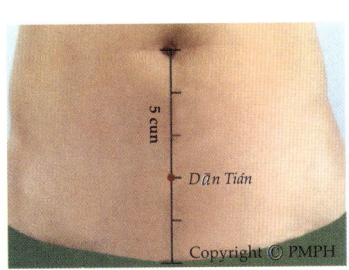

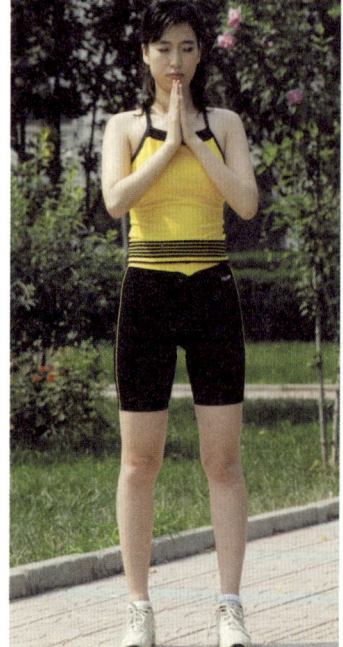
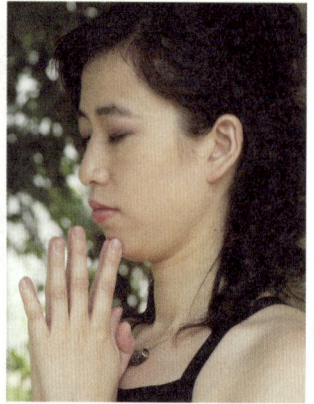

2) *Chéng jiāng* rubbing

Put the index fingers of both hands together and press gently on the point *chéng jiāng* (RN 24) with the tips of both middle fingers. Rub circularly 18-36 times clockwise and 18-36 times counterclockwise. Press the point and exhale. Release the pressure and inhale. Exhale and inhale three times and then lower both hands naturally. This is done to relieve the symptoms of dry mouth and thirst. The name *chéng jiāng* means "holding the liquid".

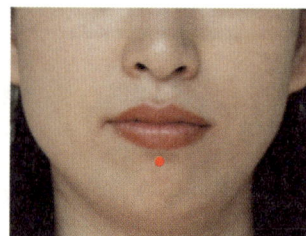
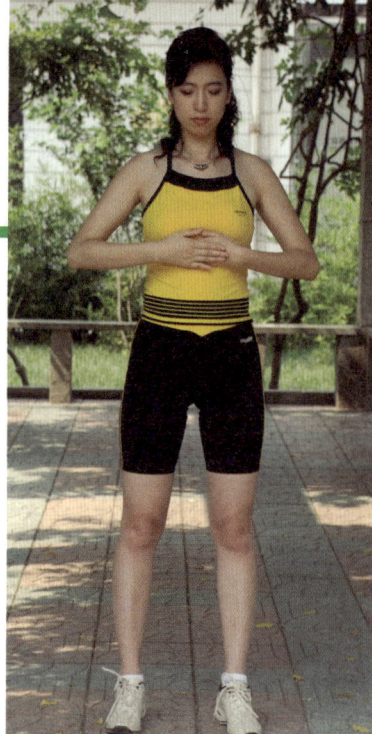

3) *Zhōng wǎn* rubbing

Put the palm of one hand on the back of the other hand and cover the point *Zhōng wǎn* (RN 12). *Zhōng wǎn* is located in the center of the abdomen, roughly 4 inches (12cm) above the belly button. Rub circularly 18-36 times clockwise and 18-36 times counterclockwise. Press the point and exhale. Release the pressure and inhale. Exhale and inhale three times. This is done to regulate the appetite. *Zhōng wǎn* means "central stomach cavity" and is a main point for strengthening the digestive organs.

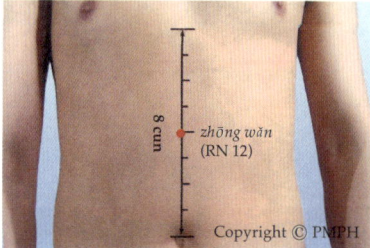

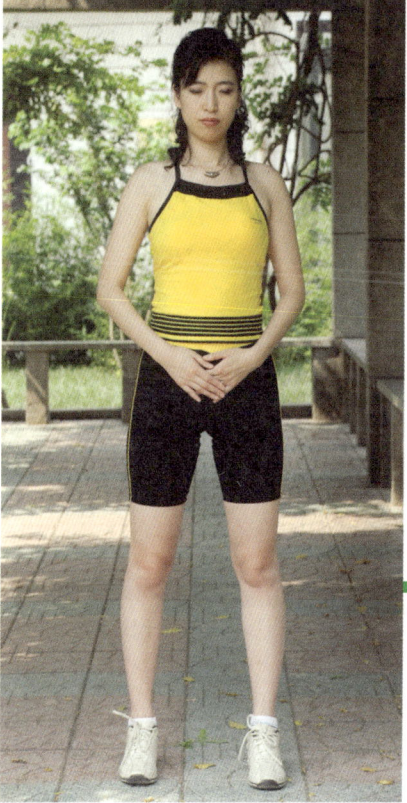

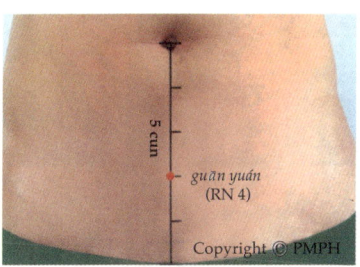

4) *Guān yuán* rubbing

Rub the point *guān yuán* (RN 4) in the same way as described above. *Guān yuán* is located on the lower abdomen, roughly 3 inches (9cm) below the belly button. This is done to supplement qi, increase energy, and to relieve the symptom of excessive urination. *Guān yuán* means "bar to the origin".

*Guān yuán is the superficial point while *dān tián* refers to the area underneath the point.

5) *Qī mén* rubbing

Put one hand on each rib side with the palms over the point *qī mén* (LR 14). *Qī mén* is located about 3 inches (9cm) below the nipple on the ribcage. Rub the point the same way as described above. This is done to regulate blood sugar levels. *Qī mén* means "cycle gate".

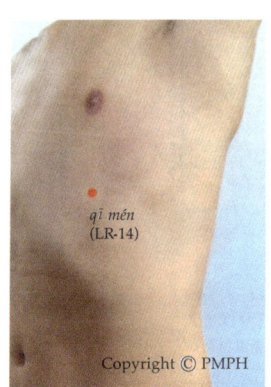

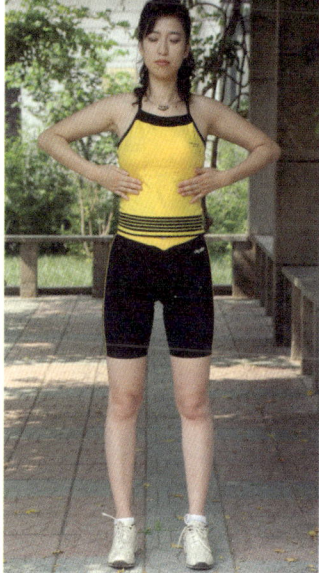

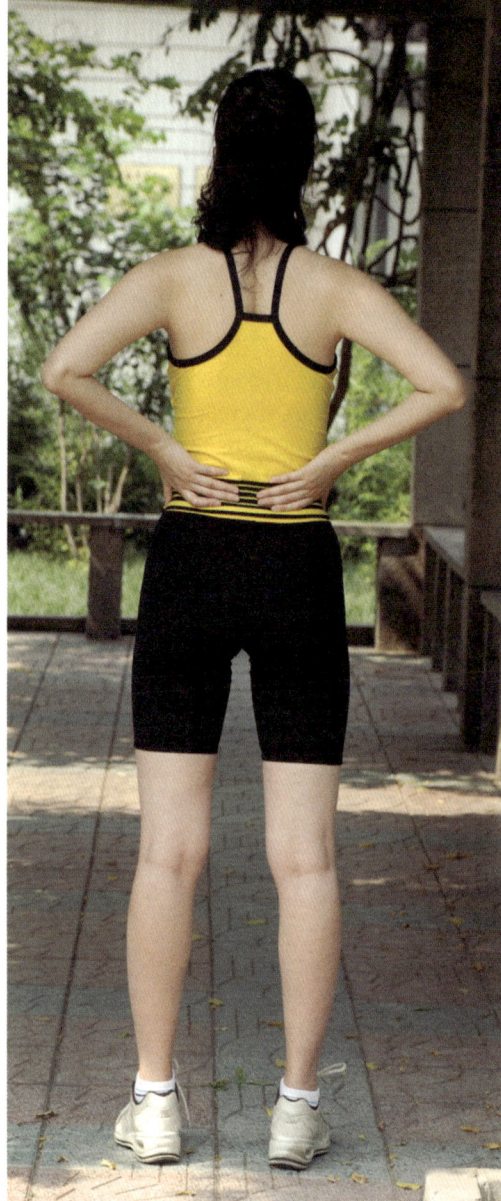

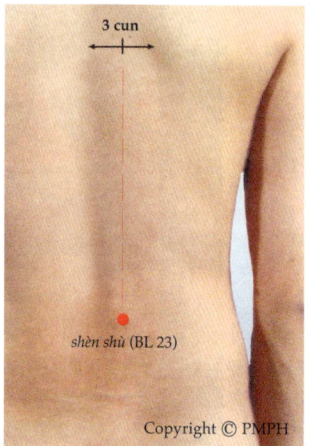

6) *Shèn shù* rubbing

Put one hand on the lower back with the palms on the point *shèn shù* (BL 23). *Shèn shù* is located on the lower back, roughly opposite the belly button, and about two finger widths from the spine. Rub the point the same way as described above. This is done to strengthen the kidney. *Shèn shù* is the transport point for the kidney.

(3) Post-massage

Do *dān tián* breathing again as described above.

This completes one round. Repeat 3 times and end by vigorously rubbing the face with your hands.

You should be calm and relaxed when giving yourself the massage. Breathe naturally from the abdomen (not shallowly from the chest). Don't hurry or make big movements and strong actions. If possible, do this routine once in the morning and once at night. One set lasts about an hour each time. It will help to relieve your symptoms, improve your body's function, and regulate blood sugar levels.

Contraindications for tui na

(1) Serious underlying diseases, such as heart, brain or lung diseases
(2) Infectious diseases like hepatitis, tuberculosis, erysipelas, or osteomyelitis
(3) Malignant tumors (other areas may be massaged)
(4) Hematological diseases with a tendency to heavy bleeding
(5) Bone fractures (other areas may be massaged)
(6) Diseased skin areas like in eczema, tinea, herpes, or scabies (other areas may be massaged)
(7) Especially weak constitution, drunk, very hungry, or full
(8) Over the abdominal and sacral regions during pregnancy or menstruation

Case 5

An 82-year-old diabetic patient received tui na therapy twice a week for 6 weeks. Before the treatment, his fasting plasma glucose, 2-hour plasma glucose, and blood lipid levels were abnormal and his blood pressure was high as well. After the treatment course, his blood sugar dropped down to normal levels and so did his blood lipid level and blood pressure. His medications (insulin and NovoNorm) were reduced.

This case is remarkable because of the age of the patient and the fact that he already suffered from many typical complications of diabetes: cataracts, coronary heart disease, a history of cerebral accidents, and diabetic nephropathy. Tui na should not be underestimated.

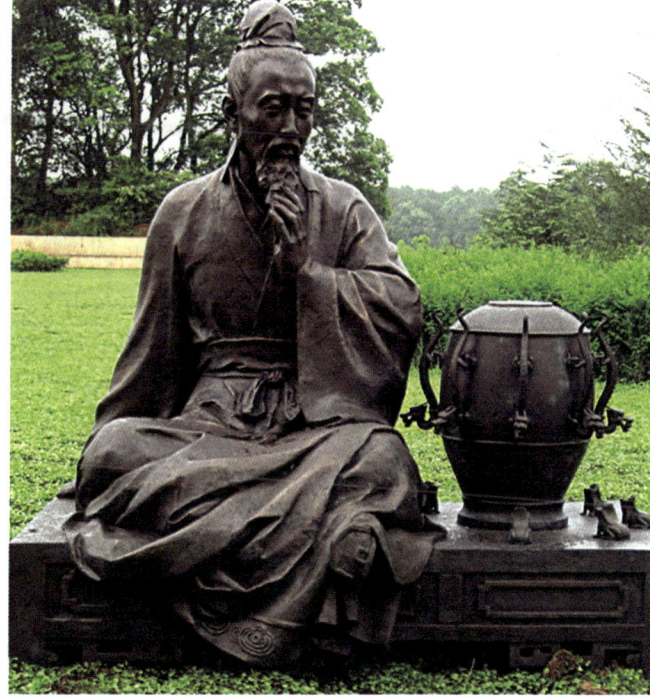

Li Shi-zhen

3. Translated Research

(1) A clinical study done in a hospital affiliated with Jinlin College of Chinese medicine found that tui na therapy can significantly lower fasting blood sugar levels and blood sugar levels 2 hours after meals in patients with type II diabetes compared with their blood sugar levels before tui na treatment. On average the fasting blood sugar went from 11.72 mmol/L (211 mg/dl) to 8.25 mmol/L (148.5 mg/dl), and the blood sugar level 2 hours after a meal went from 16.58 mmol/L (298.4 mg/dl) to 10.37 mmol/L (186.66 mg/dl). No control group was used in this study.

(2) A study on tui na done in the No.1 People's Hospital of Shanghai observed the effect of tui na combined with biomedical treatment on 237 patients with type II diabetes with a control group of 219 patients who received biomedical treatment only. The effective rate of the tui na group (who received biomedical drugs at the same time) was 89.5% while that of the control group was 78.5% (effective rate: more than 10% drop of fasting blood sugar levels, blood sugar levels 2 hours after meals, and glycated hemoglobin levels).

(3) A study done in Shandong, China, investigated the effect of tui na on fasting blood glucose and sugar tolerance of patients with type II diabetes mellitus. Thirty-eight patients with type II diabetes mellitus were selected from the outpatient clinic of the hospital affiliated to the Medical College of Qingdao University between March 2000 and March 2003. The patients were randomly divided into a treatment group and a control group with 19 cases in each group. Patients in the treatment group took Phenformin for one week and then received tui na massage therapy for 30 days. Patients in the control group orally took Phenformin for 30 days three times a day with 1-2 tablets each time. Results show that tui na massage has great efficacy on type II diabetes

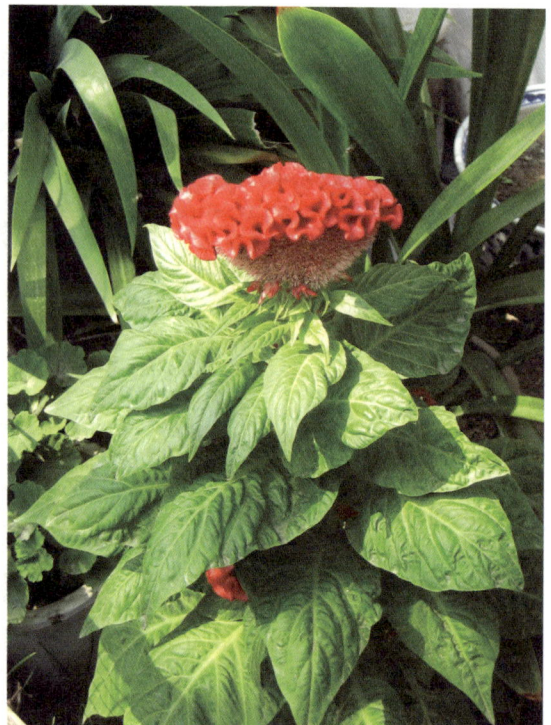

mellitus, and its short-term efficacy is significantly superior to that of Phenformin.

(4) A study in Hunan reported 72 cases of type II diabetes treated with tui na with a total effective rate of 89% (symptoms relieved, medication reduce to half or stopped, fasting blood sugar level less than 8.3mmol/L (150mg/dl), 2h blood sugar level less than 10.0mmol/L (180mg/dl), urine sugar less than 25.9g/24h or blood/urine sugar reduced more than 10%).

(5) A study done in Shanxi, China, observed the effect of tui na on diabetic peripheral neuropathy combined with biomedicine, compared to a control group that only used biomedicine. Results show that tui na plus biomedicine is significantly more effective than biomedicine alone.

(6) A study done in Hangzhou, China, compared the effect of foot bath treatment against foot bath plus foot massage on 98 cases of diabetic peripheral neuropathy. The cases were randomly divided into a foot bath group and a foot bath plus foot massage group. The two groups were also taking medication for diabetes. After a month, results showed that foot baths plus foot massage can significantly improve the symptoms of diabetic peripheral neuropathy compared with foot baths alone.

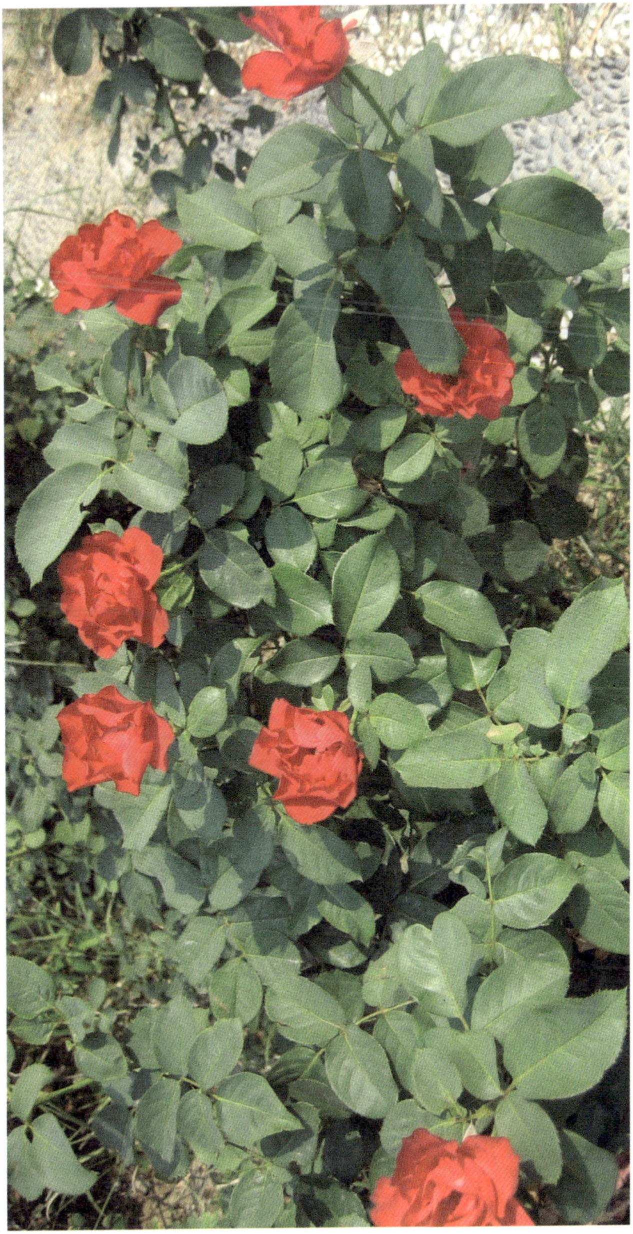

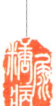

At Home Therapies

Apart from the treatment methods mentioned above, there are other simple therapies which can be done at home with the guidance of a practitioner. These therapies include hand, ear, and foot massage and foot baths. All of these therapies are based on the holistic view of Chinese medicine, together with channel theory and modern holographic theory. Holographic therapies on the hands and feet are commonly known as reflexology. These techniques work on the idea that the larger image (macrocosm) of the body is reflected on smaller images (microcosms) like the hands, feet, or ears. Treatment on the microcosm can be therapeutic for the larger body (macrocosm).

Basic theory of reflexology:

1. There are reflex points (or areas) on various holographic units in the body, such as the feet, hands, ears, etc.

2. If the function of an organ in the body becomes abnormal, there will be also abnormal signs which can be detected on the corresponding reflex area.

3. In turn, working on the reflex point (area) can also help to adjust the function of the related organ and the body as a whole to put it back to balance.

From the *jing luo* (channel theory) point of view, all the organs have correspondence points on the feet. There are 33 points below ankle on each foot. And 6 meridians originate from the feet as well.

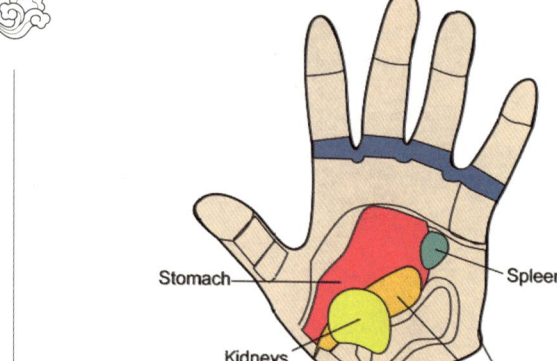
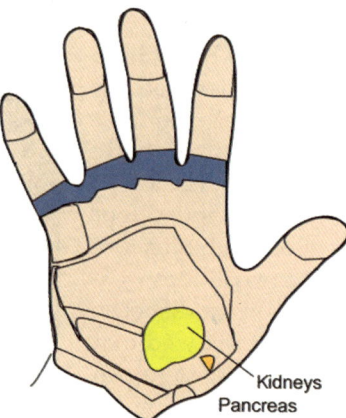

Figure 4-1 Hand Reflexology Points

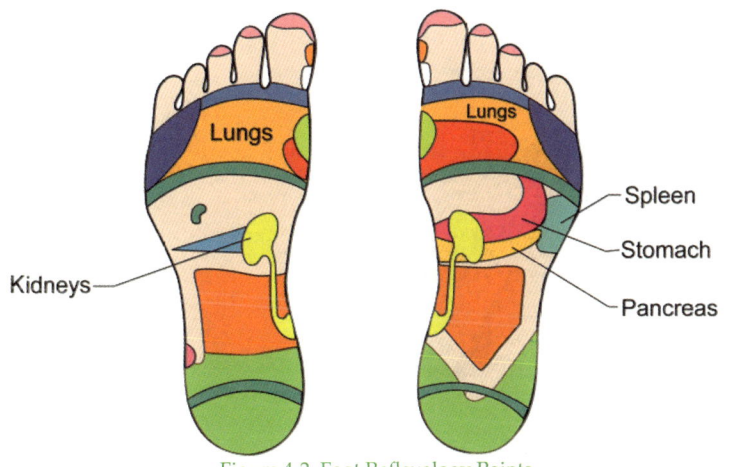

Figure 4-2 Foot Reflexology Points

By stimulating the reflex points on the hands, ears, or feet, the internal organs can be stimulated and regulated. So by stimulating the pancreas area, your pancreas will be activated. You can do this at home by yourself or with the help of a friend or family member.

Hand, Ear, and Foot Self-Massage

Gentle self-massage of the hands, ears, and feet can be done by people of all ages and conditions—children, adults, the elderly, the sick—anywhere and with or without lotion. Calming music may be used during the massage. With just a five to ten minute massage you can feel relaxed and relieved. You can follow the procedure recommended here, or that recommended by your practitioner.

Pre-massage

Wash your hands, face, and feet with warm water. Play light music if you like. Sit comfortably. Relax yourself and empty your mind. You can also use lotion on your hands, especially if your skin is dry.

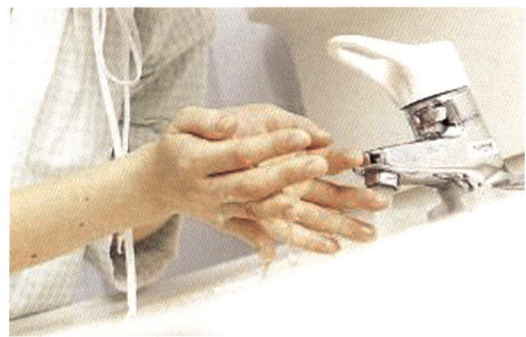

(1) Hand Massage

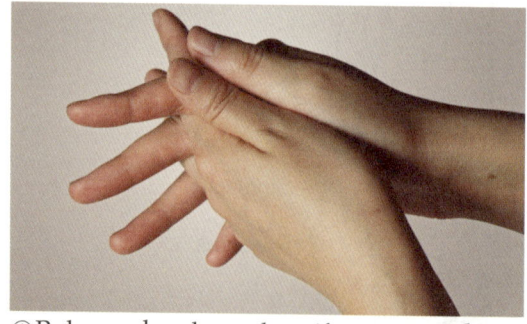

①Rub your hands gently as if you are washing them.

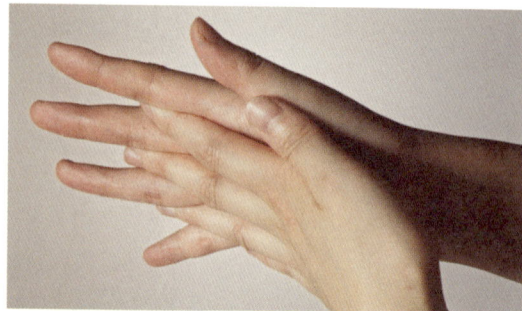

②Open the palm of your hand with the other one, gently pressing the palm and stretching the muscles of the hand.

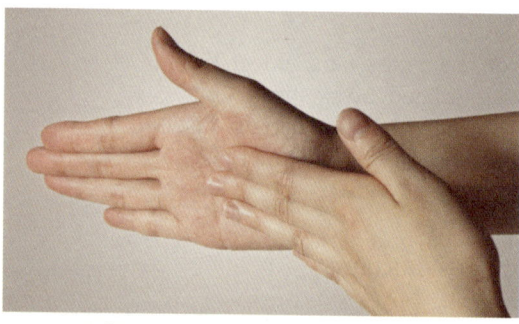

③Press the reflexology points shown on the above illustration.(See Figure 4-1)

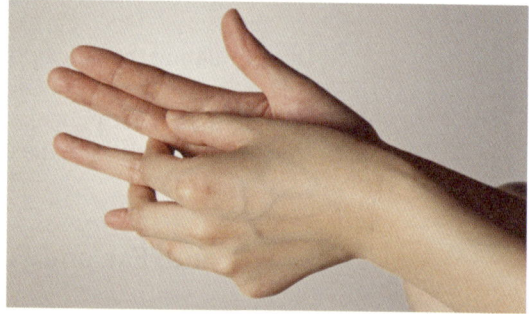

④Massage the muscles and tendons between the bones of the hand.

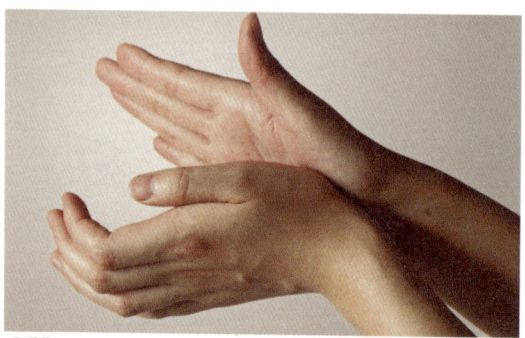

⑤Use your wrist to massage the opposite palm.

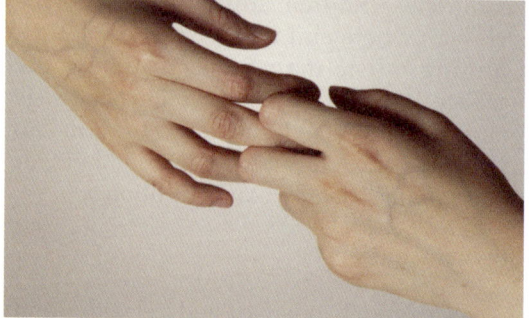

⑥Massage each finger and pull the fingers, visualizing the tension pouring out of the fingertips.

(2) Ear Massage

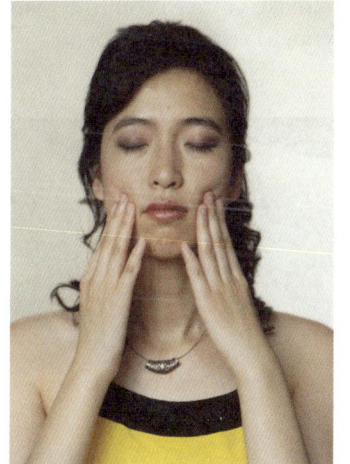 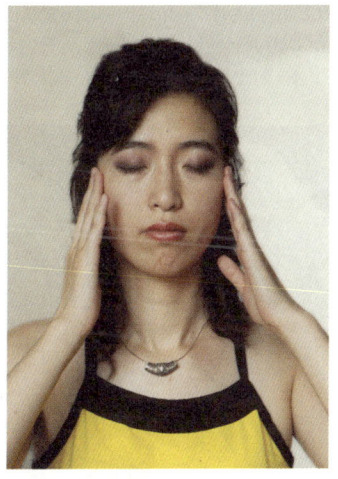 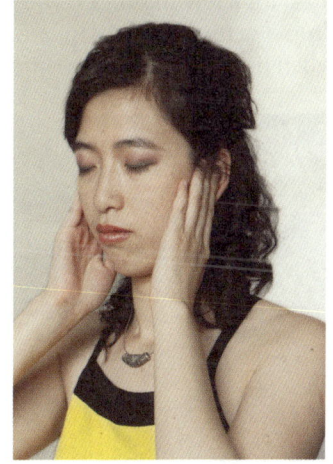

① Massage your face with your finger tips from jaw to cheeks using gentle, circular motions. Widen the circle to touch the ears.

②Massage your ears all over and warm them with your hands.

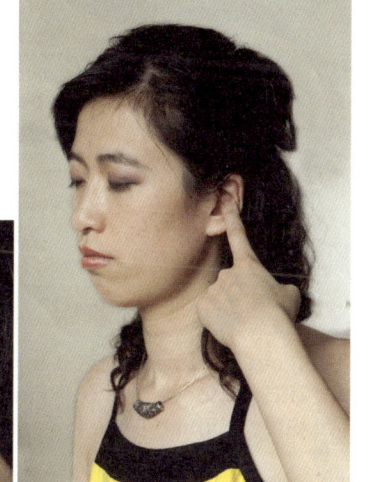 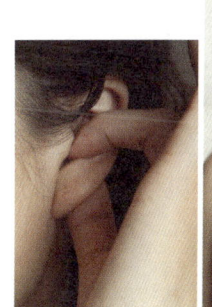 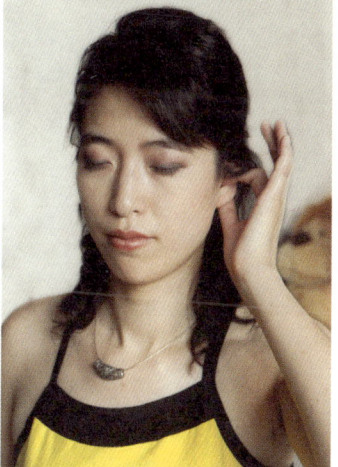

③Stretch the lobes gently and press the reflexology points shown on the image of Page 82.

(3) Foot Massage

*Rest for a few minutes if you are feeling tired. Adjust your position to make yourself comfortable. Prop one foot in your lap and let the other rest extended in front of you. Massage one foot and when finished, change position and do another.

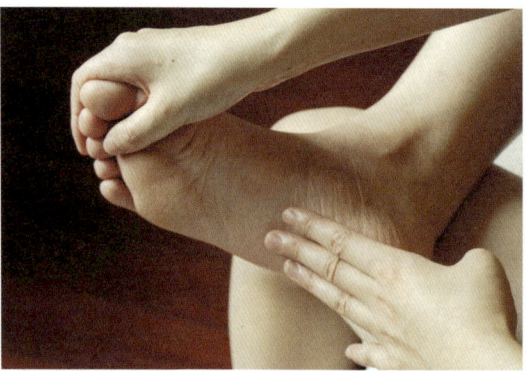

① Put one hand on top of the foot and the other closer to your toes, then stroke smoothly from your toes to your ankles.

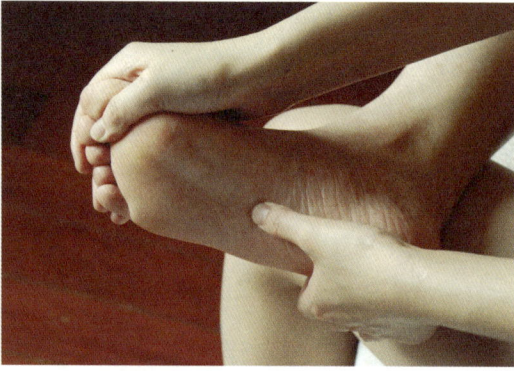

② Glide your hands to the sole of your foot and massage the reflexology points shown in the image.

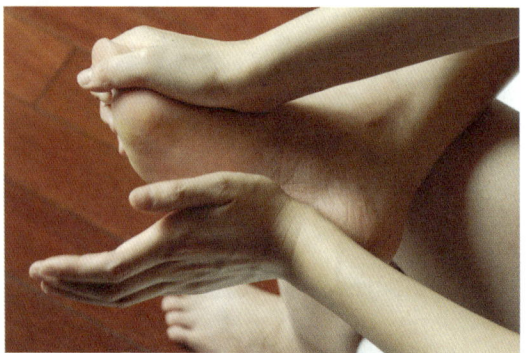

③ Press the arch of the foot with your wrist.

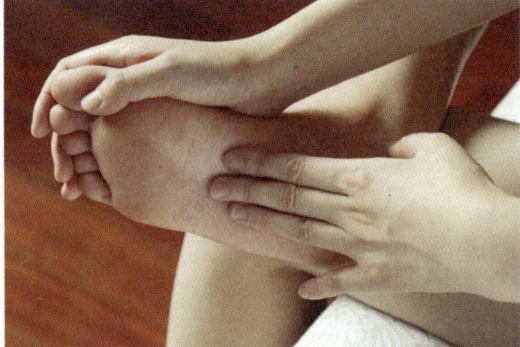

④ Again put one hand on top of the foot and the other closer to your toes, then stroke smoothly from your toes to your ankles.

You can do the above procedure every other day or twice a week. In a month you will feel better. Continue to massage yourself regularly to ensure a lasting effect.

Foot fumigation or foot bath

Foot fumigation or foot bath refers to therapies that use a warm medicinal decoction to bathe or fumigate the feet. It is used to prevent or treat peripheral vascular complications, especially diabetic neuropathy of the feet. The warmth combined with the medicinals act on the feet to benefit the flow of qi and blood. The ingredients of the decoction should be given by your practitioner based on your specific pattern identification. Herbs that can move blood and remove stasis are often used to promote local circulation and metabolism. In addition, herbs that supplement qi and yin and open the channels are often used to treat the root condition. A lot of research showing the effectiveness of medicinal foot baths has been done.

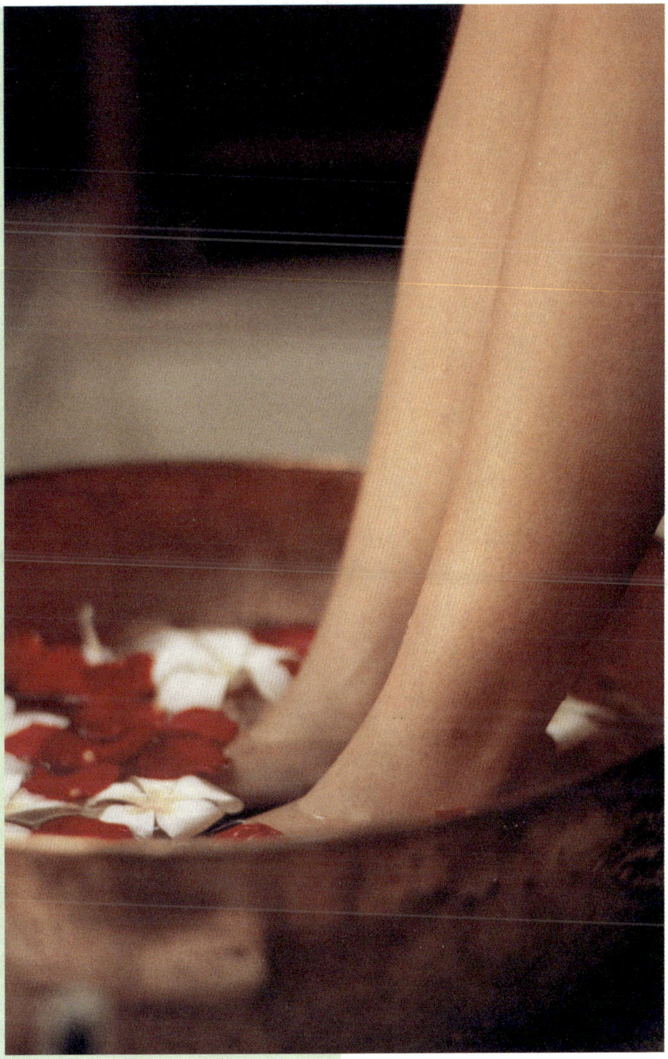

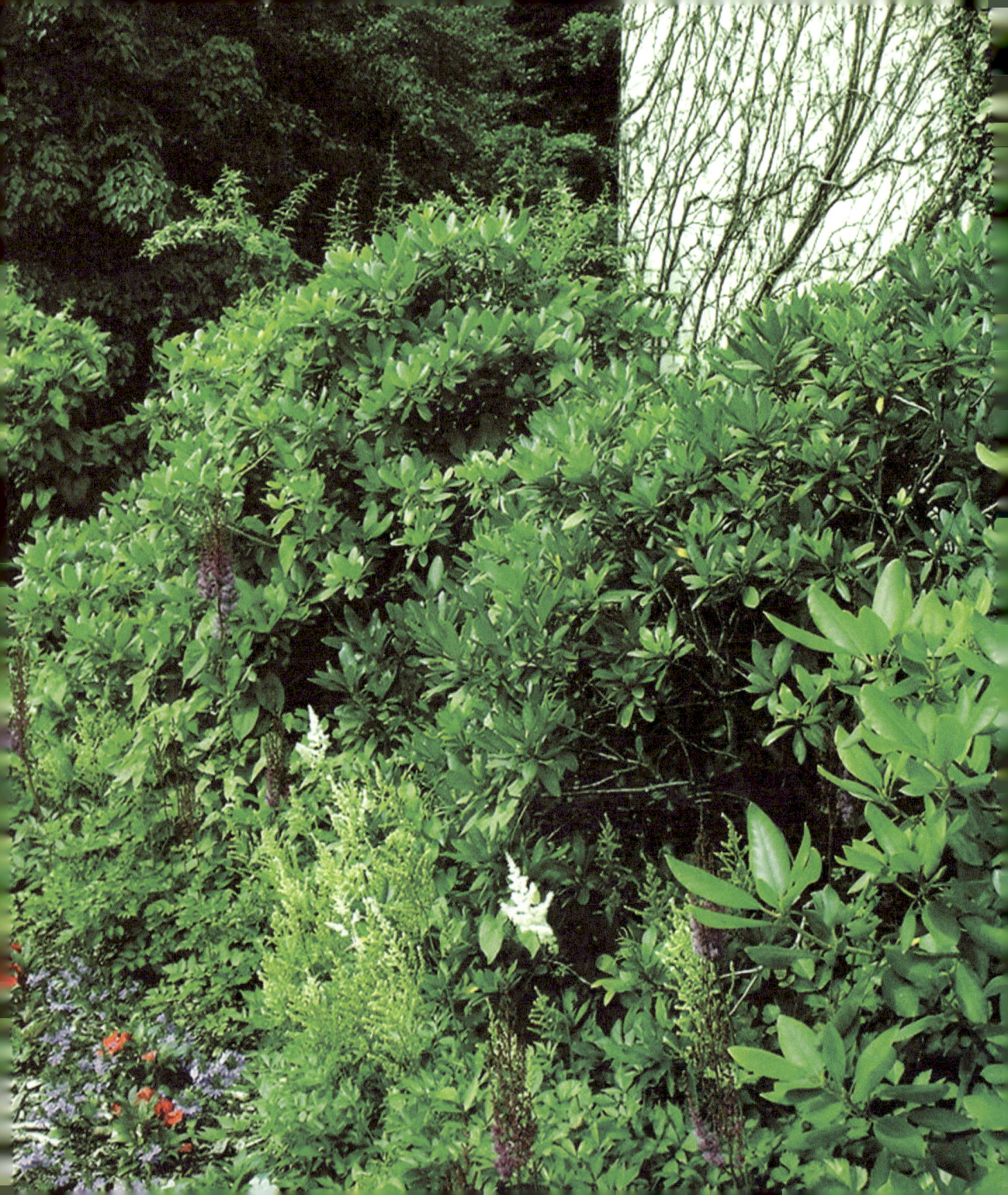

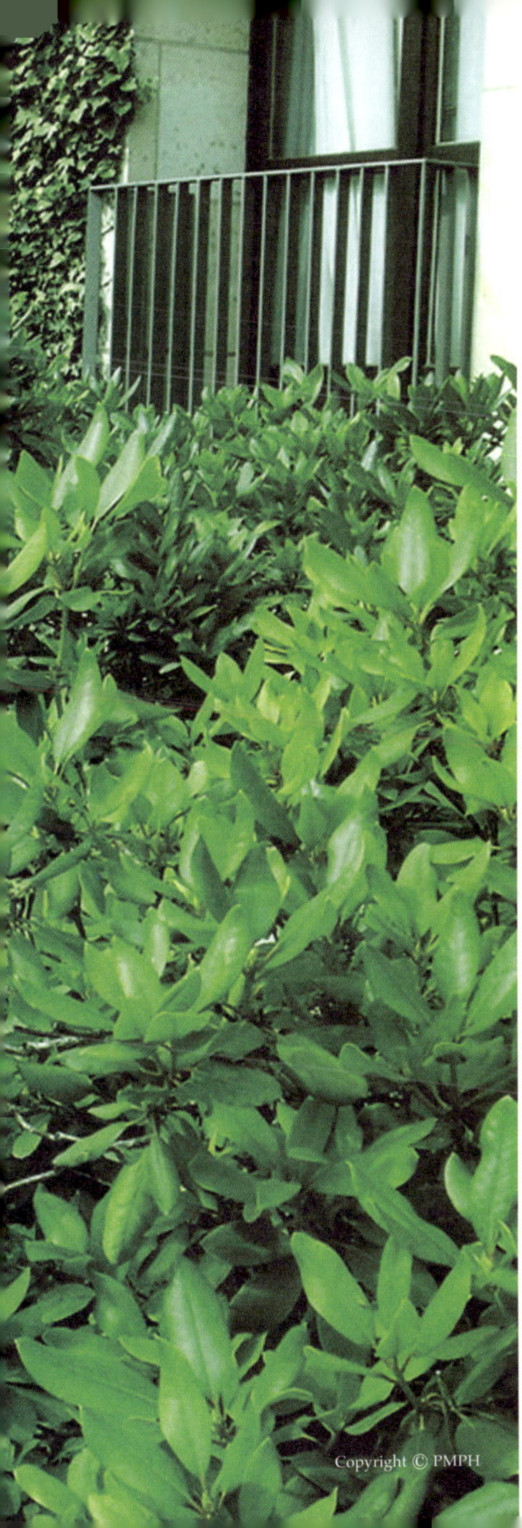

Chapter 5

Case Studies

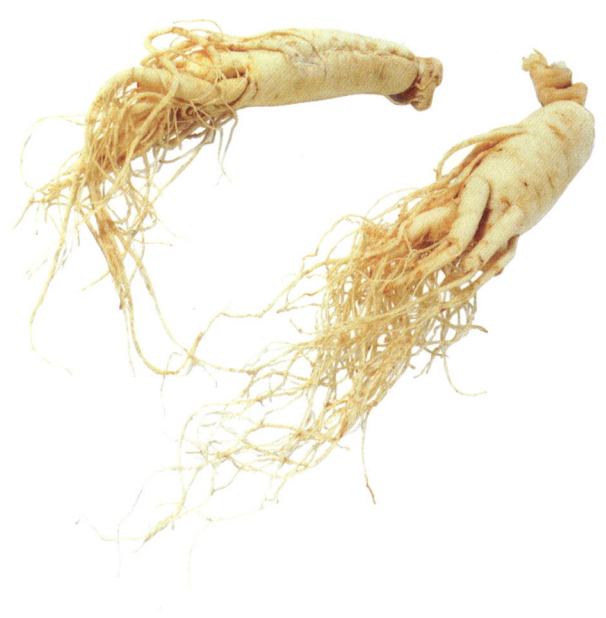

This final chapter includes various case histories from real patients with diabetes. They represent the standard of care for diabetes patients with Chinese medicine. As you have seen above, diabetes has been rigorously studied both in the clinic and the laboratory. These cases are to show you that by using this knowledge, real people have been able to bring their disease under control and lead healthy lives. You may notice that nearly all the histories involve treatment with herbal medicine, usually prescribed to be taken as a decoction every day for a number of weeks or months. For those who were initially attracted to treatment with Chinese medicine because of what they heard about acupuncture, we encourage you to give herbal medicine a fair trial. It is the most effective, safest, and fastest way to health with Chinese medicine.

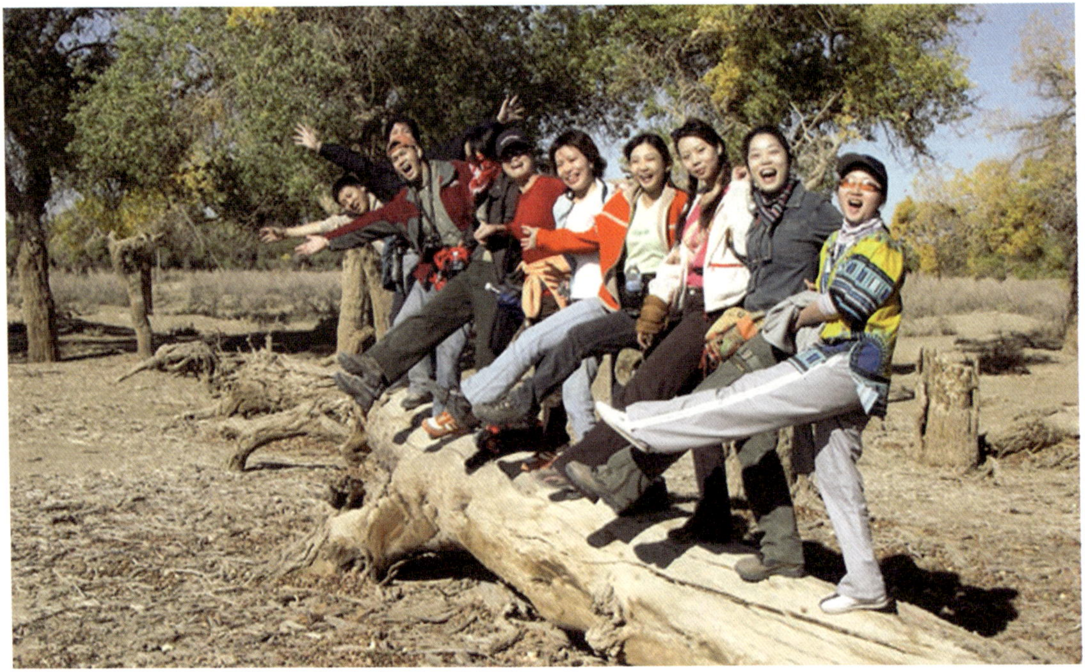

You are about to read case histories of patients with type II diabetes mellitus. All of them are seeking treatment from natural medicine in addition to biomedical treatment. These accounts might not be totally unfamiliar, and from reading this book, you will be able to understand something about the Chinese medical theory and treatment protocols.

Case 1

Mr. Hua, aged 46, works as a social service worker and is married with one son. He is well built but seldom exercises. A sedentary lifestyle and heavy diet have given him a belly. He smokes (15 cigarettes per day on average) and drinks alcohol (150-200ml per day on average) and has done so for over 20 years. He has always been fairly healthy except for the occasional common cold.

At the age of 41 during a routine check-up, Mr. Hua was found to have elevated blood sugar levels. He didn't think too much of it at the time because he felt quite well most of the time. Occasionally he was a bit tired, which he attributed to aging. Several months later, however, he suddenly felt fatigued and nauseous with blurred vision after drinking too much at a social gathering. He went to the hospital immediately and was diagnosed with diabetic ketoacidosis. His blood sugar had reached 27.3 mmol/L (491.4 mg/dl) with a large amount of ketones in the urine. After he recovered and was released from the hospital, he was diagnosed with type II diabetes and put on pharmaceutical medication.

Figure 5-1 Lab Result

First Name:	xxx	Gender:	Male
Last Name:	Hua	Age:	41
Fasting Plasma Glucose:		27.3mmol/L	

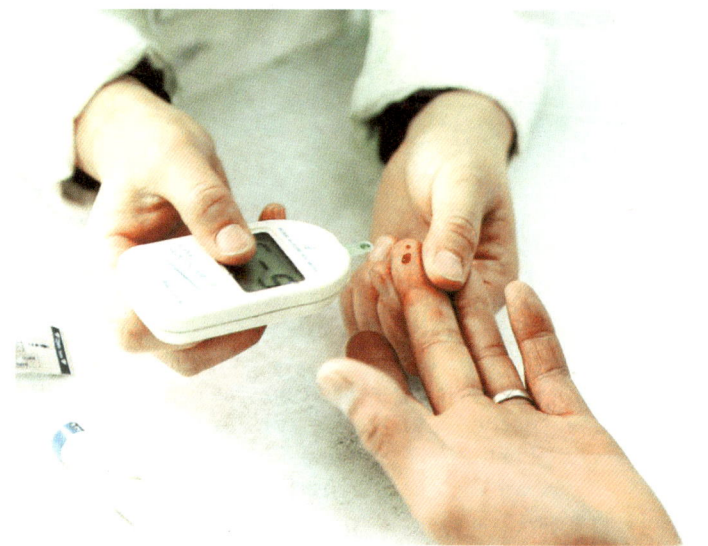

After leaving the hospital, Mr. Hua didn't pay much attention to his condition. He thought he could still live the way he did if he took his medication regularly. He didn't watch his blood sugar or restrict his diet. Several complications and hospitalizations followed after which Mr. Hua decided to be more careful with his diet and lifestyle. Despite following the doctor's advice and taking his medication, his condition continued to deteriorate and he felt fatigued and very worried.

On a recommendation from his friend he went to consult a practitioner of Chinese medicine.

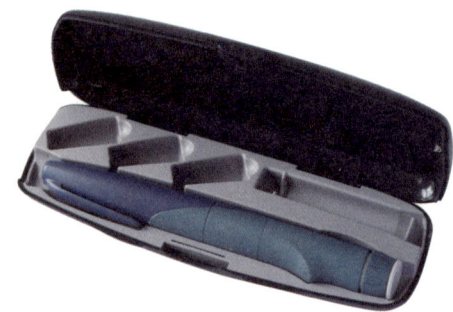

An Insulin Injector

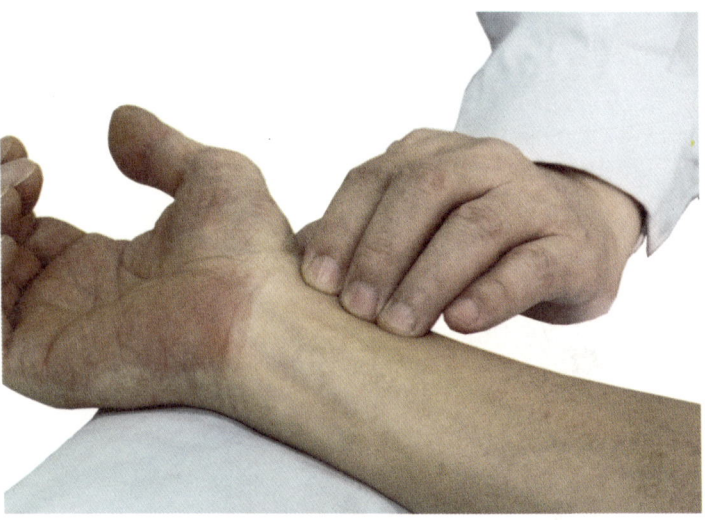

At the clinic the practitioner performed a detailed inquiry and physical exam just like any biomedical doctor would. The difference was an extra tongue inspection and careful pulse examination. The diagnosis of Mr. Hua in Chinese medical terms was: *Xiao ke bing* (disease of emaciation and thirst), qi deficiency and blood stasis.

The cause of the disease was seen as Mr. Hua's unhealthy lifestyle leading to an imbalance of qi, blood, yin and yang. In Mr. Hua's case, the qi, weakened by years of poor health management, is failing to promote the flow of blood. Herbs were prescribed to regulate the body's function so as to improve insulin resistance and allow his general condition to improve.

He was also put on a restricted diet and given an exercise regimen to follow. Since Mr. Hua's pattern was qi deficiency and blood stasis, the treatment methods were selected to strengthen qi and promote the flow of blood.

Mr. Hua was given one packet of herbs to boil per day. At first, the doctor supplied three days worth of herbs, and adjusted the prescription frequently. During this time, Mr. Hua continued to take biomedical drugs for his disease.

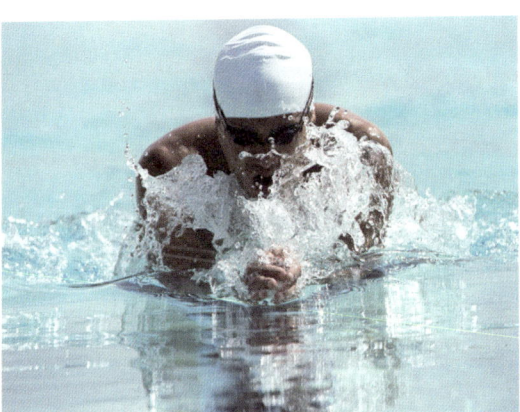
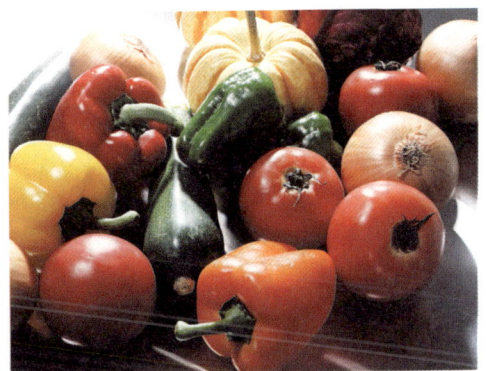

After three weeks of treatment Mr. Hua's blood sugar became stable. And equally important, he felt more energetic and had a rosy complexion. His blood pressure returned to normal and he no longer felt fatigued. Mr. Hua was very pleased. He was warned, however, that he needed to continue treatment for a while in order to consolidate the effect of the treatment. For type II diabetes patients, lifestyle modification must be combined with any treatment given. Only using integrated methods can diabetes be controlled.

Eventually, the practitioner gave Mr. Hua a 14-day dose of herbs and asked him to come back for a follow-up two weeks later to adjust the formula if necessary.

Mr. Hua continued an integrated treatment with Chinese medicine and biomedical drugs together with dietary and lifestyle changes. Generally speaking, he feels a sense of well-being. Occasionally, when he feels unwell or catches a cold, he goes to a Chinese medicine practitioner to regulate his condition. He feels good and his condition is stable without any complications or emergency flare-ups.

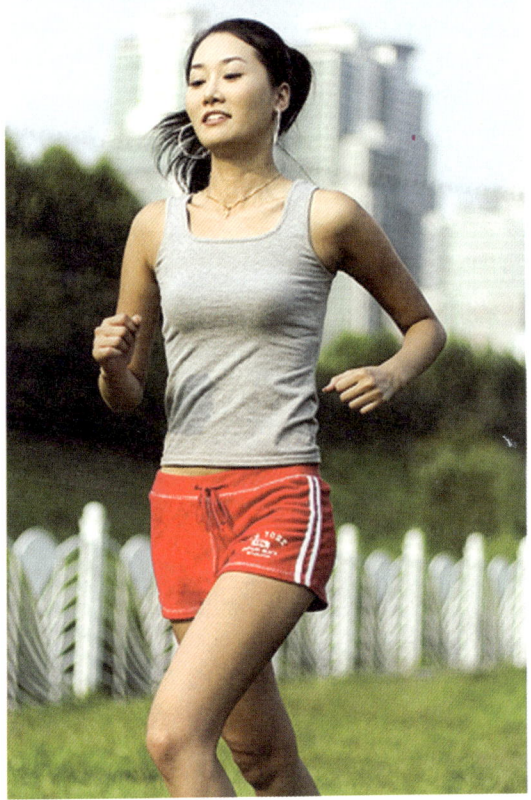

Case 2

Mr. Li, a 61 year old man, was a successful executive and had a history of good health. When he first came to the clinic he complained of an unquenchable thirst and soreness and weakness in the lower back and knees for the past three years. About the time the symptoms started he was diagnosed with diabetes while in for a routine check-up. He was treated with Gilemal and a prepared pill of Chinese medicinals, but still his blood sugar was not controlled and the above symptoms began to get worse. He also suffered from an increased appetite, fatigue, and dry stool. His complexion was reddish and his tongue was dark red with a thin, yellow, and slightly greasy coating. His pulse was fine and slippery. The lab tests revealed blood glucose at 13.0mmol/L (234 mg/dl). According to the signs and symptoms Mr. Li was diagnosed with qi and yin deficiency due to stomach heat. A Chinese medicinal prescription was given, which Mr. Li boiled for himself every day.

Table 5-1 Prescription for Mr. Li

Medicinal name	Pinyin	Dose	Latin name
Trichosanthin	tiān huā fěn	25g	Radix Trichosanthis
Kudzuvine Root	gě gēn	25g	Radix Puerariae Lobatae
Common Anemarrhena Rhizome	zhī mǔ	15g	Rhizoma Anemarrhenae
Golden Thread	huáng lián	10g	Rhizoma Coptidis
Rehmannia Dride Rhizome	shēng dì huáng	25g	Radix Rehmanniae Recens
Figwort Root	xuán shēn	25g	Radix Scrophulariae
Common Yan Rhizome	shān yào	15g	Rhizoma Dioscoreae
Danshen Root	dān shēn	15g	Radix et Rhizoma Salviae Miltiorrhizae
Evonymus Alata	guǐ jiàn yǔ	15g	Lignum Suberalatum Evonymi
Lychee Seed	lì zhī hé	15g	Semen Litchi
Hairyvein Agrimonia Herd	xiān hè cǎo	30g	Herba Agrimoniae

He took this formula for a month. One packet of herbs boiled every day.

The patient was also advised to change his diet, maintain regular physical activity, and keep a calm mind.

On the second visit a month later his thirst was relieved and he had more physical energy. His bowel movements also became easier. The same formula was given for another month. On the third visit he no longer felt thirst or soreness and weakness in the lower back and knees. His tongue coating looked normal and his pulse was fine. His glucose levels were down to 9.8mmol/L (176.4 mg/dl). This formula was continued for another two months where his glucose eventually reached 6.9mmol/L (124.2 mg/dl). And he felt great. After four months of cooking herbs for himself, Mr. Li was given a formula to take long term in pill form.

A follow-up three years later showed good health and normal lab results.

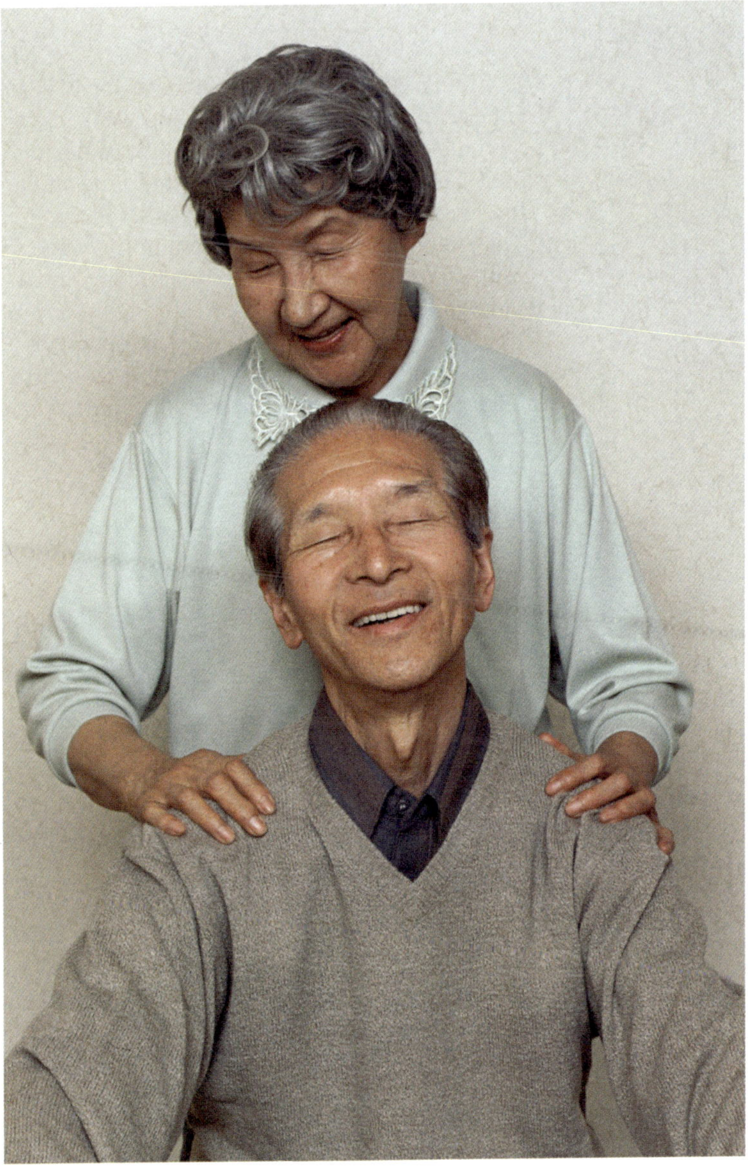

Case 3

Mr. Zhang, 60, suffered from diabetes for 10 years. He complained of edema in both legs and feeling weak. He also felt dizzy, had no appetite, slept poorly, sweated at night, and had to urinate 3-5 times per night. He had a dark-red colored tongue and a yellowish greasy coating. His pulse was deep and weak. He had high blood glucose levels as well as glucose and protein in his urine. He took Enalapril three times a day, Diamicron two times a day, and a prepared Chinese medicinal pill three times a day.

He decided to try professional treatment with Chinese medicine. The practitioner he visited thought he would be helped by both acupuncture and herbal medicine and suggested a treatment program for the next three months.

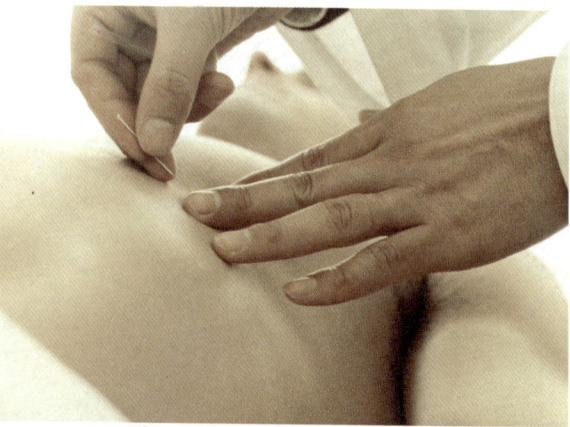
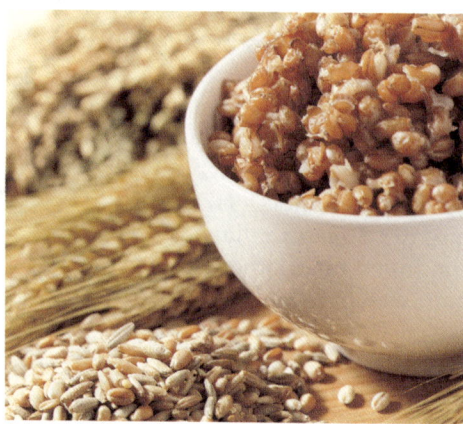

Acupuncture treatments were done once every other day. Each session lasted about 30 minutes. Mr. Zhang also was given herbs to boil and drink every day. After three months of treatment, his dizziness and edema were gone, as were his night sweats. He still got up to urinate at night, but only once or twice, otherwise he slept well. His lab test results had also improved.

Case 4

Ms. Weng, 58, first visited the clinic in May of 1998. She had suffered from diabetes for eight years, taking a prepared Chinese medicinal pill (*Xiaoke* pill) and metformin at the same time, but her blood sugar levels were not under control. She complained of weakness, shortness of breath, sweating, restlessness, irritability, a strong thirst, constipation, numbness in the limbs, and burning heat in the soles of the feet. Her tongue was red with little coating and her pulse was fine and rapid. She was diagnosed with deficiency of qi and yin. The doctor prescribed a formula containing Radix Scrophulariae (*xuán shēn*), Radix Puerariae Lobatae (*gě gēn*), Radix Rehmanniae Recens (*shēng dì huáng*), and other herbs to boost qi and nourish yin. After two months of treatment her condition had stabilized. Her symptoms were mostly gone and her blood sugar was much lower. In a follow-up visit six months later she remained healthy.

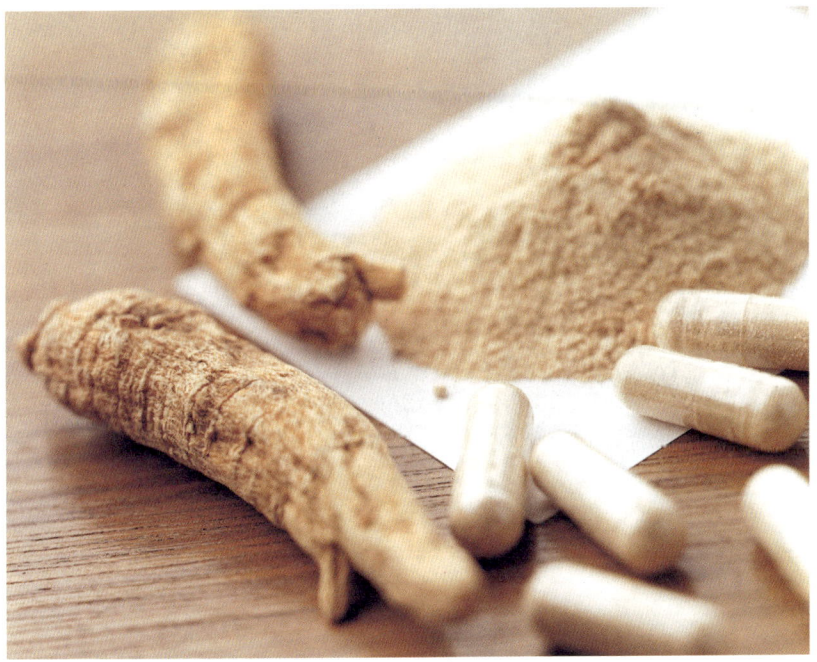

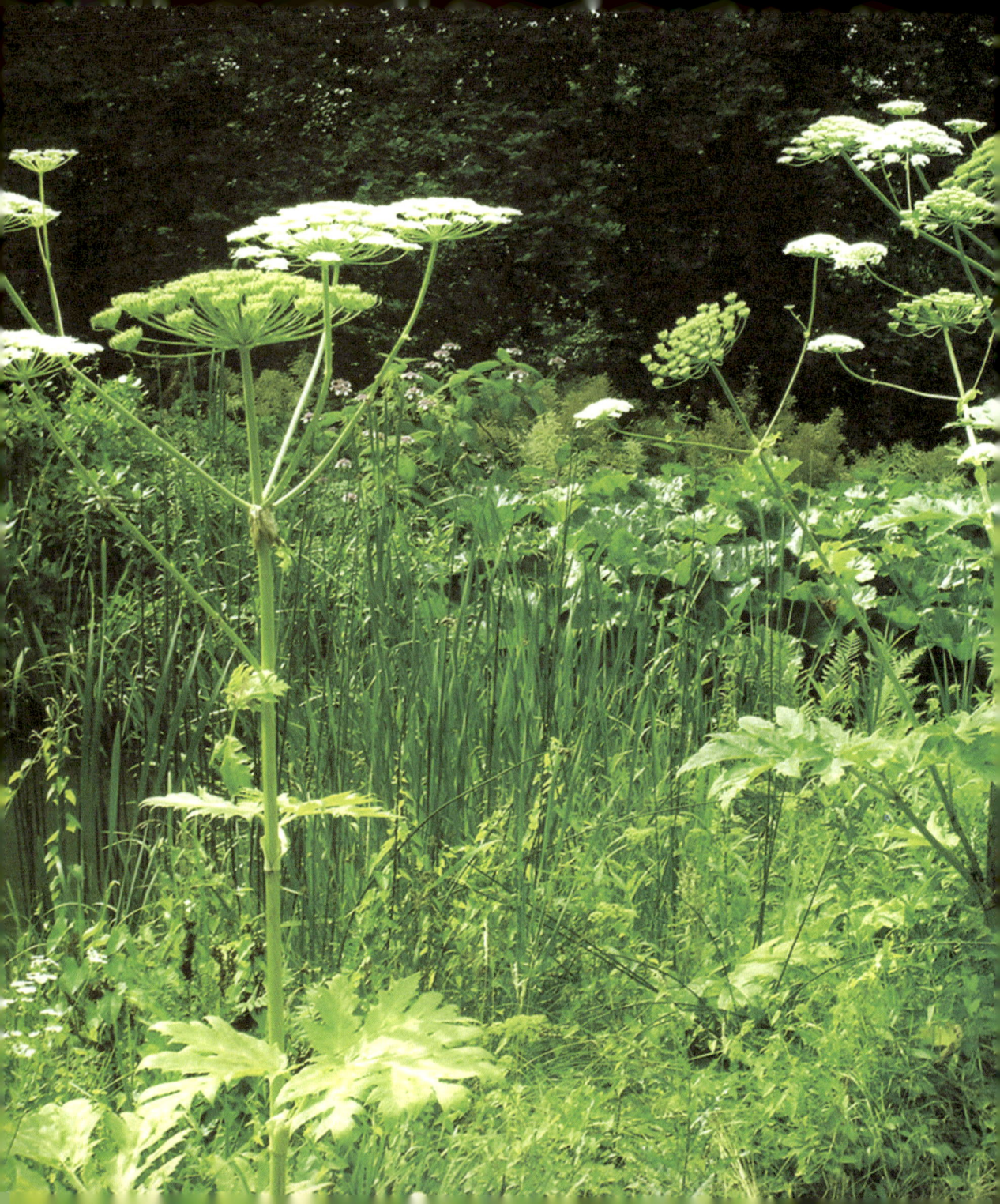

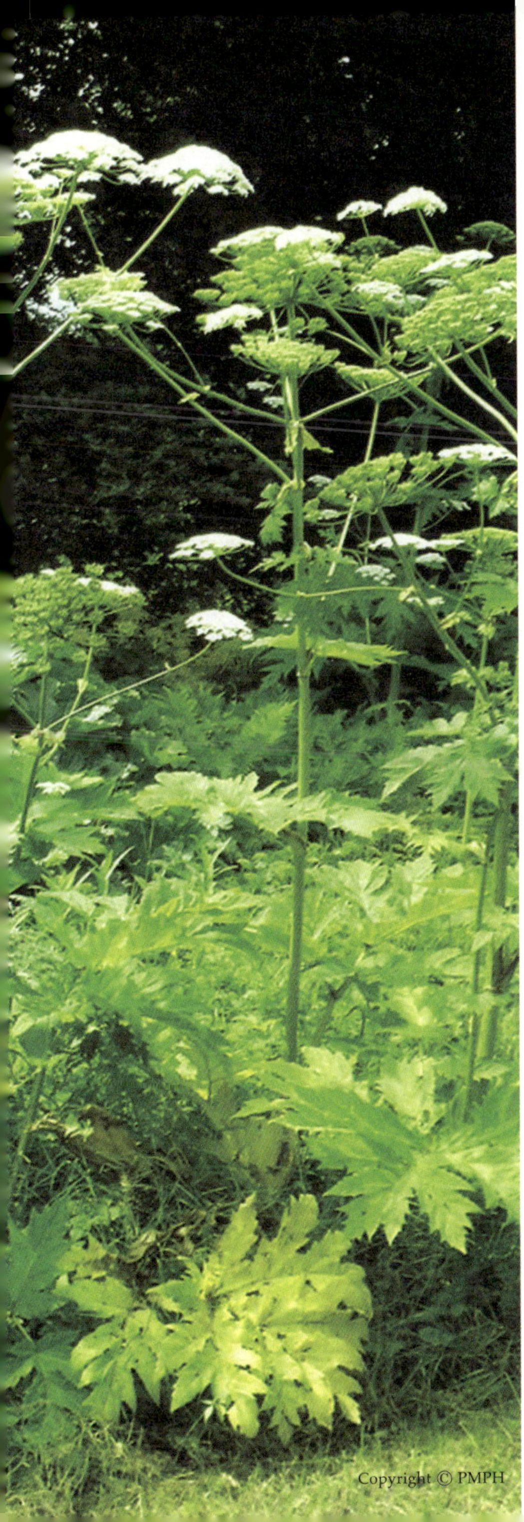

Conclusion

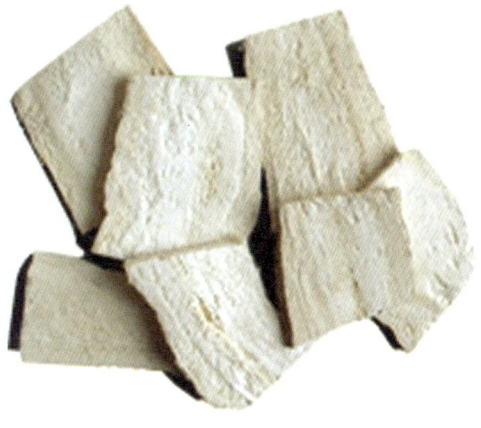

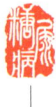

We hope this book has given you another option when it comes to managing your health.

Chinese medicine is not a magic pill, nor is biomedicine. Each system studies the amazing human body in its own way, with its own philosophy. Biomedicine sees the human body as a machine and analyzes each part in fantastic detail. Its strength is its precision and accuracy. Eventually, it will have the entire human body mapped out in the greatest detail. A doctor's job is to nail down the exact part that is broken down and fix it. The question for a doctor is: What is wrong? As a patient, it is difficult to understand much about your treatments as biomedicine is extremely technical and there are so many details.

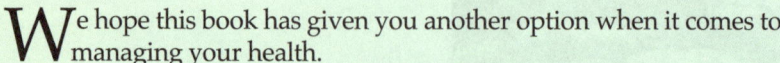

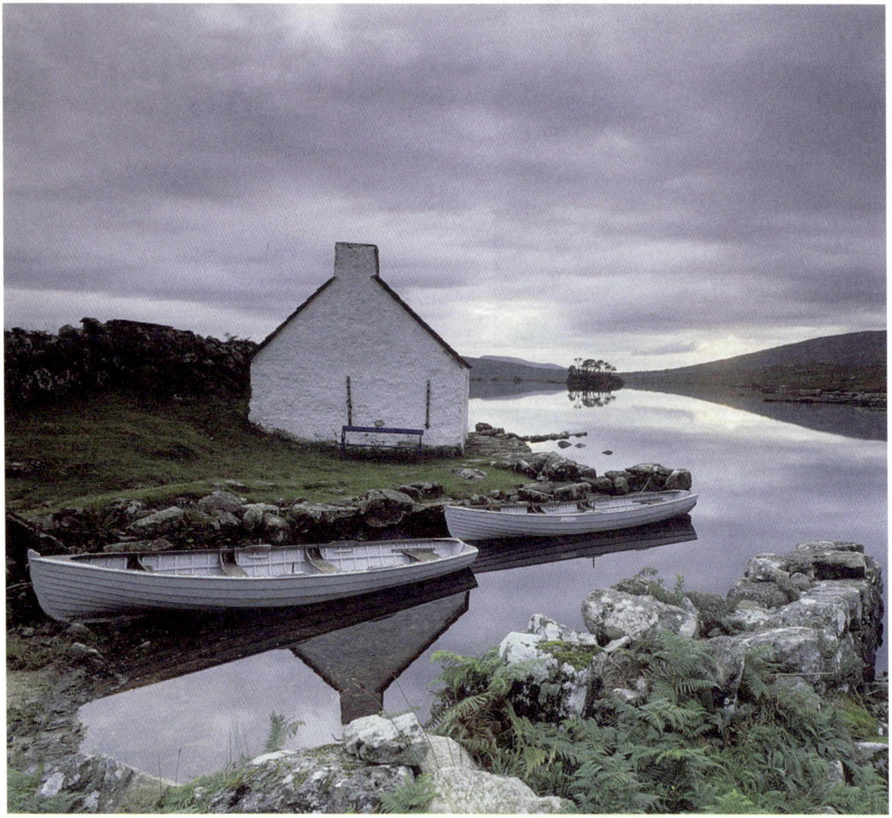

Meanwhile, Chinese medicine sketches a figure that is inseparable from his complex surroundings. In Chinese medicine, a human is neither a jigsaw puzzle nor a machine, but like a tree growing in soil, a fish swimming in water, or a bird flying in the sky. When it comes to accuracy and precision, Chinese medicine might not compare to biomedicine. Its strength is seeing the big picture. A practitioner's job is to evaluate the patient's general condition and find where the imbalances lie. As a patient, you may not have the training to evaluate your own imbalances of yin and yang, but you have the ability to understand what is wrong, and more importantly, how you can act to restore health.

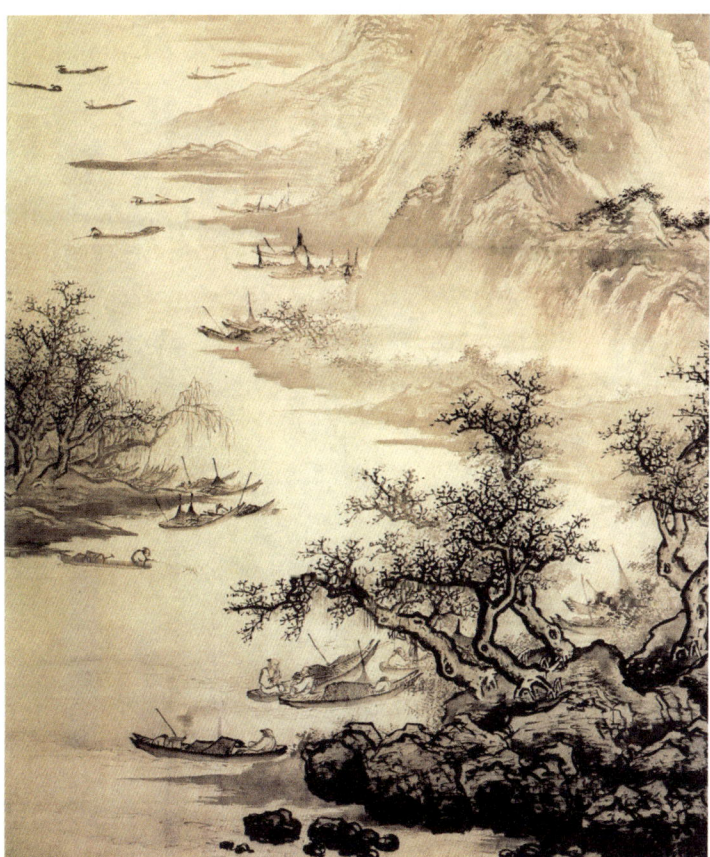

In the future these two medicines will be integrated to benefit all mankind. It will take time. It will take understanding. Most of all, it will take wisdom, the wisdom to eliminate inhibition and choose freedom, the wisdom to judge which choice is best.

Get the medicine you need, no matter eastern or western.

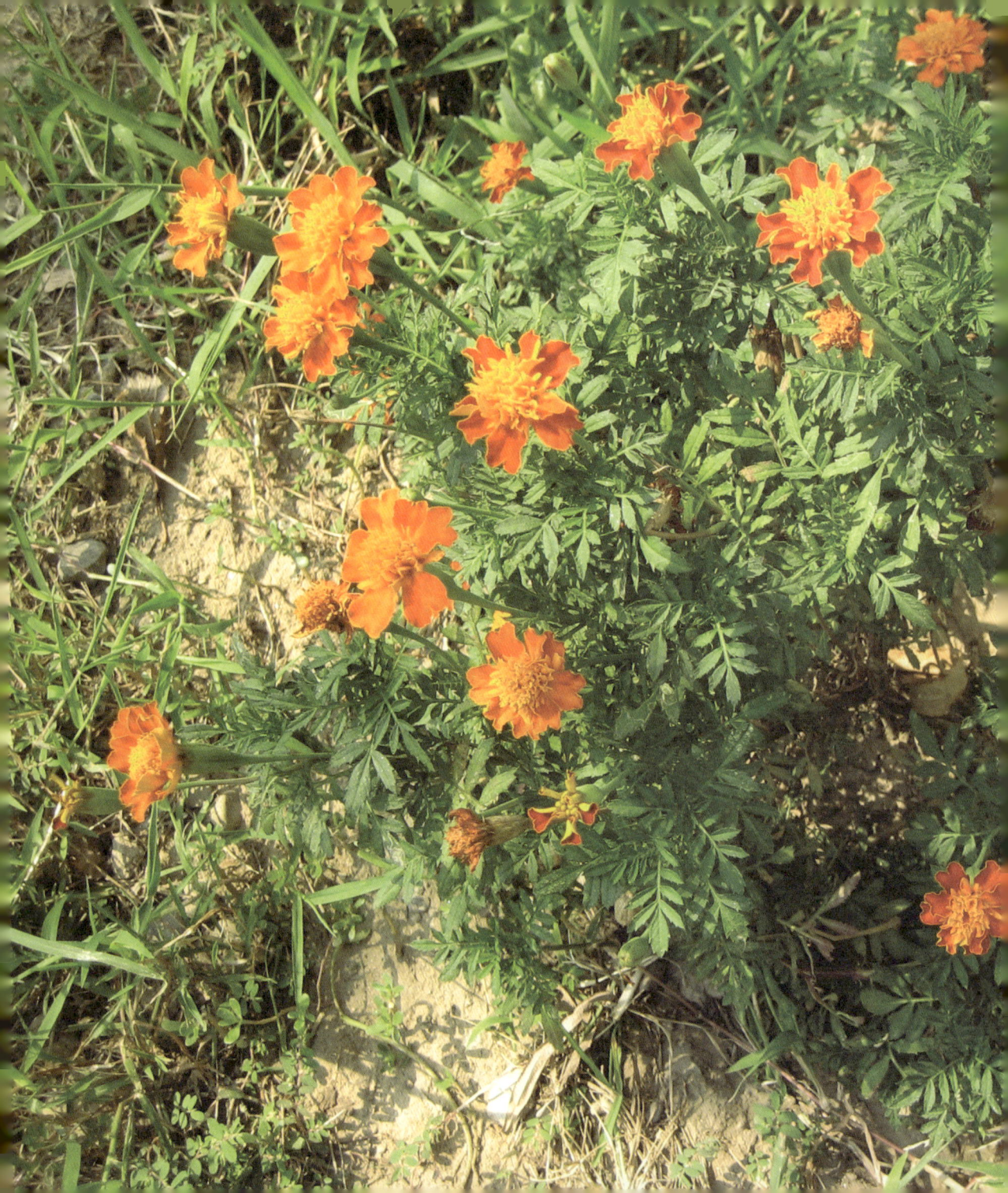

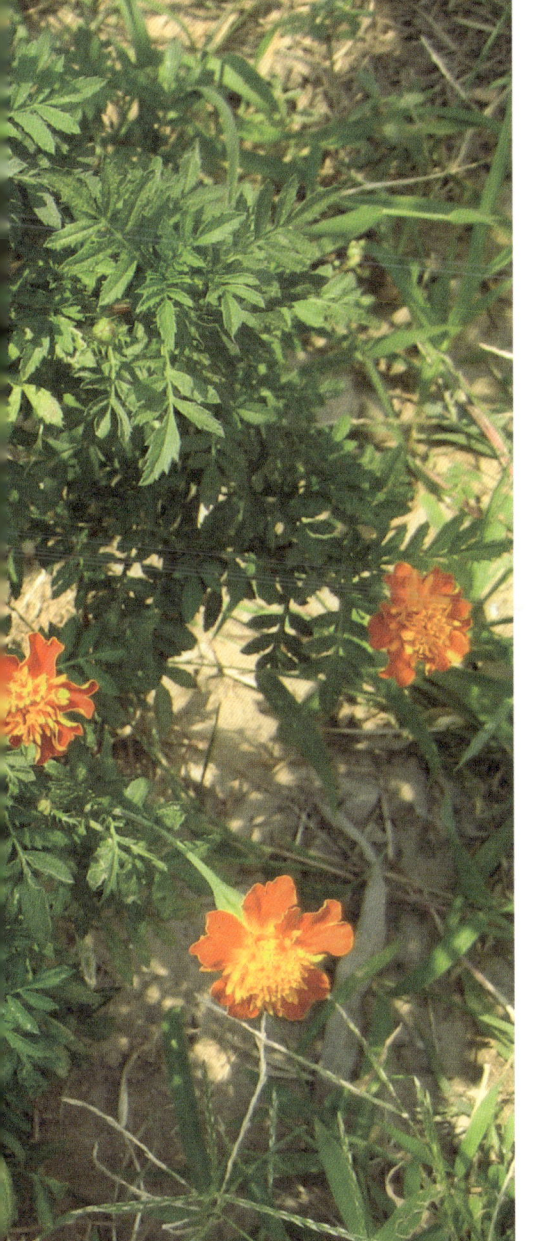

Appendix

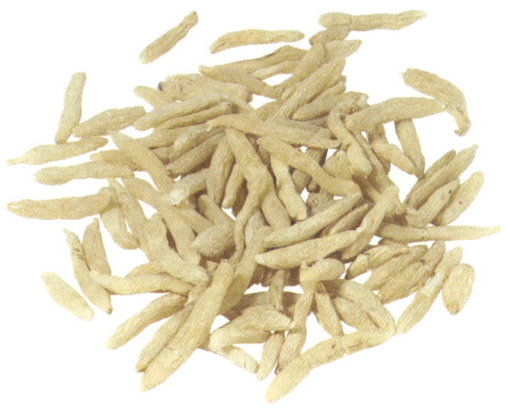

1. Basic Disease Information (Biomedicine)

> Adapted from Diagnosis and Classification of Diabetes Mellitus. American Diabetes Association. Diabetes Care, Volume 30, Supplement 1, January 2007

Basic information

Diabetes mellitus results from problems in insulin secretion, insulin action, or both, which cause hyperglycemia. Chronic hyperglycemia will cause damage and dysfunction to the eyes, kidneys, nerves, heart, and blood vessels.

The typical symptoms of hyperglycemia include frequent urination, a strong thirst, weight loss (sometimes in spite of increased food intake), and blurred vision. Failure to heal from injuries and increased susceptibility to infections may also be present. Acute, life-threatening consequences of uncontrolled hyperglycemia are ketoacidosis or the nonketotic hyperosmolar syndrome.

Long-term complications of diabetes include retinopathy with risk of loss of vision; kidney problems leading to renal failure; peripheral neuropathy with risk of foot ulcers and amputations; and autonomic nervous system problems causing gastrointestinal, urinary, cardiovascular, and sexual dysfunction. Patients with diabetes are at risk for atherosclerosis, peripheral arterial disease, and cerebrovascular accidents. Hypertension and high cholesterol are also problems for diabetes patients.

Table 7-1 Classification of Diabetes

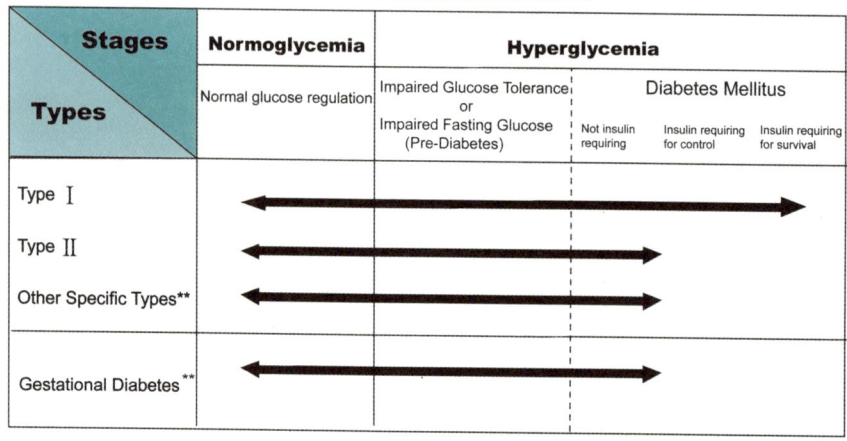

Disorders of glycemia: etiologic types and stages. *Even after presenting in ketoacidosis, these patients can briefly return to normoglycemia without requiring continuous therapy (i.e., "honeymoon remission");
rare instances, patients in these categories (e.g., Vacor toxicity, type 1 diabetes presenting in pregnancy) may require insulin for survival.

Table 7-2 Criteria for the Diagnosis of Diabetes Mellitus

> 1. Symptoms of diabetes plus casual plasma glucose concentration ≥200 mg/dl (11.1mmol/L) Casual is defined as any time of day without regard to time since last meal. The classic symptoms of diabetes include polyuria, ploydipsia, and unexplained weight loss.
> OR
> 2. FPG ≥126mg/dl (7.0mmol/L). Fasting is defined as no caloric intake for at least 8 h.
> OR
> 3. 2-h postload glucose ≥200mg/dl (11.1mmol/L) during an OGTT. The test should be performed as described by WHO, using a glucose load containing the equivalent of 75g anhydrous glucose dissolved in water.
>
> In the absence of unequivocal hyperglycemia, these criteria should be confirmed by repeat testing on a different day. The third measure (OGTT) is not recommended for routine clinical use.

There is a third stage which lies between a non-diabetic and the diagnosis of full diabetes. This is when a patient's lab tests fall into an area which is labeled impaired glucose tolerance (IGT) or impaired fasting glucose (IFG). These levels are defined as having fasting plasma glucose (FPG) levels over 100 mg/dl (5.6 mmol/L) but under 126 mg/dl (7.0 mmol/L) *or* 2-h values in the oral glucose tolerance test (OGTT) of over 140 mg/dl (7.8 mmol/L) but under 200 mg/dl (11.1 mmol/L).

Thus, the categories of FPG values are as follows:
- FPG less than 100 mg/dl (5.6 mmol/L) is normal fasting glucose;
- FPG between 100 and 125 mg/dl (5.6–6.9 mmol/L) is IFG (impaired fasting glucose);
- FPG over 126 mg/dl (7.0 mmol/L) is provisional diagnosis of diabetes (the diagnosis must be confirmed).

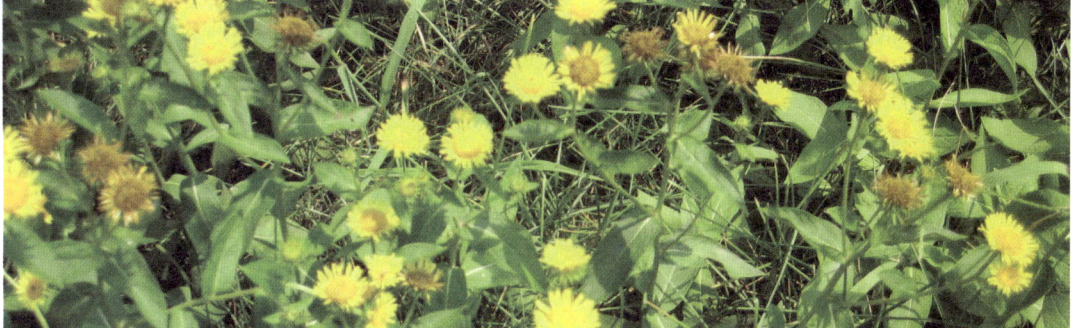

2. Global/National Statistics

A Global Diabetes Mellitus Epidemic

Statistics taken from the web page of the International Diabetes Federation www.idf.org. Diabetes Atlas, third edition International Diabetes Federation, 2006

Diabetes, mostly type II, now affects nearly 6% of the world's adult population with almost 80% of the total in developing countries. The number of people with diabetes mellitus is expected to increase alarmingly in the coming decades. In 1985, an estimated 30 million people worldwide had diabetes; in 2000, a little over a decade later, the figure had risen to over 150 million. In 2007, the figure is expected to shoot up to 246 million and continue rise to 380 million by 2025 if no urgent action is taken.

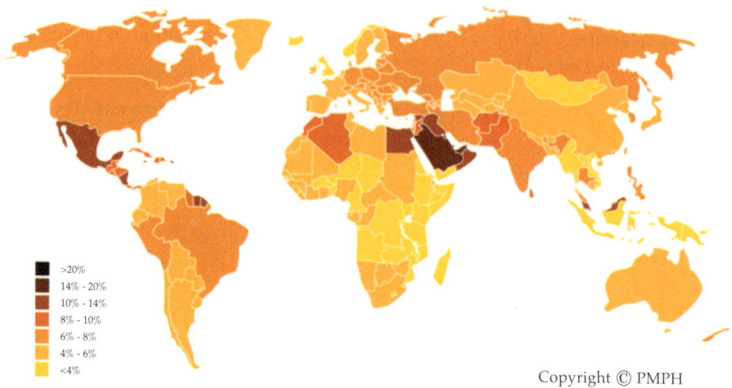

Figure 7-1 Source: Diabetes Atlas Third Edition, International Diabetes Federation, 2006

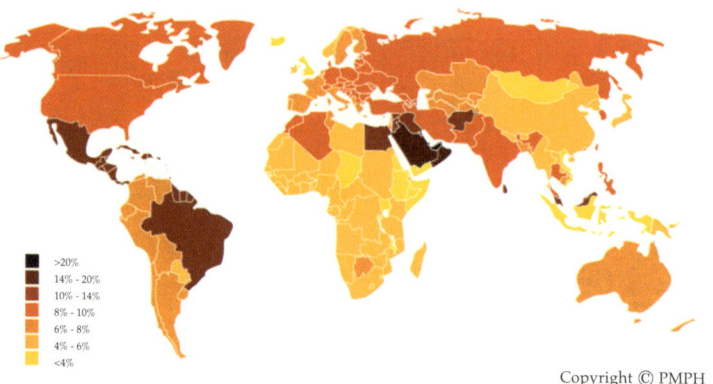

Figure 7-2 Source: Diabetes Atlas Third Edition, International Diabetes Federation, 2006

The regions with the highest rates are the Eastern Mediterranean and Middle East, where 9.2% of the adult population is affected, and North America (8.4%). The highest numbers, however, are found in the Western Pacific, where some 67 million people have diabetes, followed by Europe with 53 million. In the US alone, 20.8 million people or 7.0% of the population has diabetes.

While developed nations are home to 80% of diabetes cases, poorer countries will be the hardest hit by the coming rise in diabetes patients. Increased urbanization, westernization and economic development in developing countries have already contributed to a substantial rise in diabetes.

With the forces of globalization and industrialization proceeding at an increasing rate, the prevalence of diabetes is predicted to increase dramatically over the next few decades. The resulting burden of complications and premature mortality will continue to present itself as a major public health problem for most countries. The diabetes "epidemic" is already upon us.

Diabetes mellitus: deadly and costly, silently haunting

We all know diabetes is a chronic non-communicable disease, but not all of us know how silent deadly and extremely costly this disease is.

To live, or not to live?

Diabetes causes about 5% of all deaths globally each year.

In 2005, 1.1 million people died from diabetes. The full impact is much larger because though people may live for years with diabetes, their cause of death is often recorded as heart diseases or kidney failure. Researchers from the World Health Organization (WHO) using a computerized disease model reported overall 2.9 million deaths in 2000 (5.2% percent of all deaths) were attributable to diabetes or complications of diabetes. Of these deaths, 1 million occurred in developing countries and 1.9 million occurred in developed nations.

The lowest proportion of deaths (2.4 percent) was seen in the poorest African countries and in Cambodia, Laos, Myanmar and Vietnam. It was highest (9 percent) in the Arabian Peninsula and the Americas (8.5 percent).

Diabetes is expected to cause 3.8 million deaths worldwide in 2007, about 6% of total global mortality, which is about the same as caused by HIV/AIDS. Using WHO figures on years of life lost per person dying of diabetes, this translates into more than 25 million years of life lost each year.

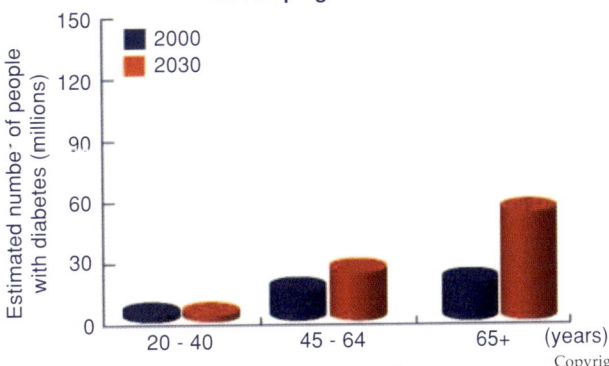

Figure 7-3 Estimated Number of Adults with Diabetes

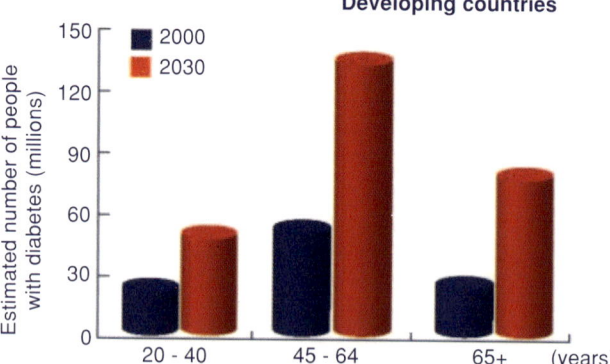

Figure 7-4 Estimated Number of Adults with Diabetes

The International Diabetes Federation (IDF) estimates that the equivalent of an additional 23 million years of life are lost to the disability and to reduced quality of life caused by the preventable complications of diabetes.

The WHO projects that diabetes deaths will increase by more than 50% in the next 10 years without urgent action. Most notably, diabetes deaths are projected to increase by over 80% in upper-middle income countries between 2006 and 2015.

To pay, or not to pay?

Diabetes affects all of society, not just those who live with diabetes. The annual direct health care costs of diabetes worldwide, for people in the 20-79 age bracket, is estimated to be at least 153 billion US dollars and may be as much as $286 billion, or even more.

If predictions of diabetes prevalence are fulfilled, total direct healthcare expenditures on diabetes worldwide will be between 213 billion and 396 billion US dollars in 2025. This would mean that the proportion of the world's health care budget being spent, in 2025, on diabetes care will be between 7% and 13% with high prevalence countries, such as Nauru, spending up to 40% of their budget.

In many countries a substantial proportion of healthcare costs are borne by the individual and the family. Estimates of the indirect cost of diabetes, i.e. the cost of lost production, are as high as direct costs or even higher than those for direct costs. In developing countries, in families where one member has diabetes treatment may cost 25% of their annual income. This puts them in the horrible position of having to choose between getting treatment and having to live in extreme poverty, or going without and living with avoidable disabilities or premature death.

By 2007, the medical expenditure on diabetes mellitus and its complications is expected to amount to somewhere between 215 to 375 billion US dollars, most of which is spent in developed countries.

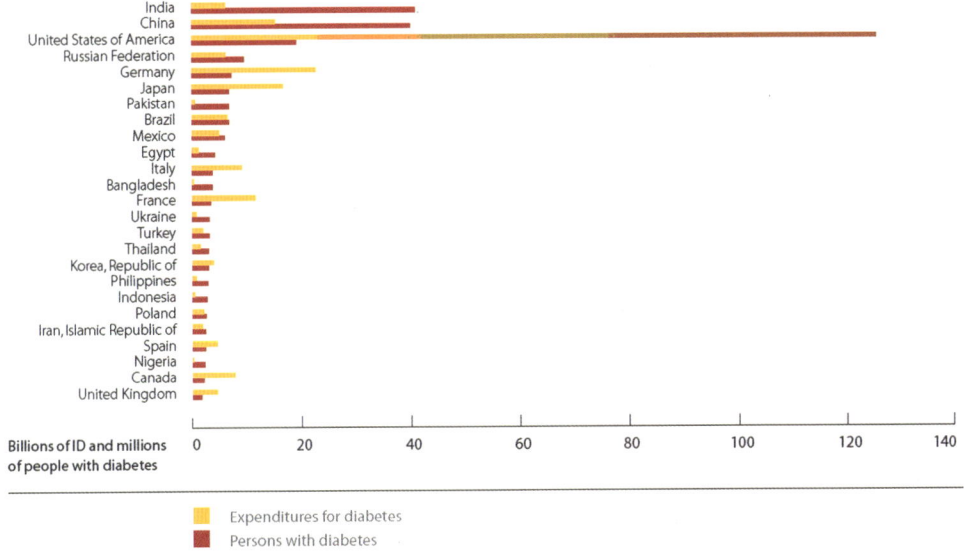

Figure 7-5 Annual Health Expenditure for Diabetes (ID) vs Persons with Diabetes in the 25 Countries with the Largest Numbers of Persons with Diabeters in 2007

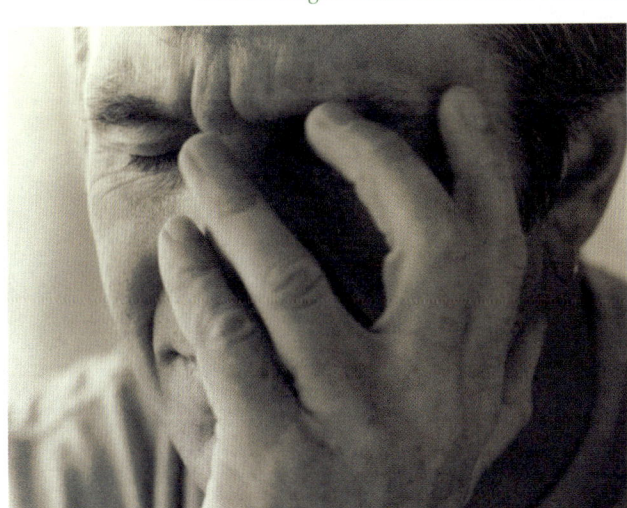

Faced with all these facts and figures, we can't deny the presence of a problem. We cannot help asking: Why? And more importantly, how to solve the problem?

> One book is not enough to answer these two questions. Politically, historically, economically and medically, there are a lot factors to be blamed in contributing to the present situation.

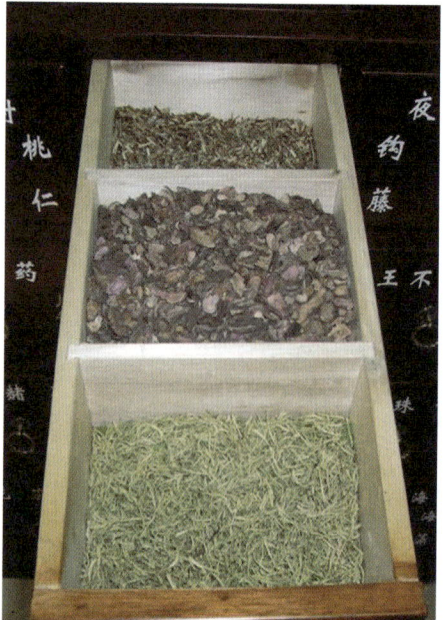

On one hand, we have a whole array of advanced medication at hand. If the pancreas is not working, we have insulin. If the body cannot use insulin properly, we have Metformin or the like. We also have new drugs coming on the way, like Januvia, newly approved by the American FDA. They all promise to lower blood sugar levels with different mechanisms. But they cannot solve the fundamental problem and they have to be consumed daily for the rest of the patient's life. With all this we are still faced with ever-increasing burdens and sufferings of diabetes mellitus.

With a lot of factors to be blamed, unhealthy diet, physical inactivity, tobacco use, insufficient education, improper stress-management, limited access to medication for the poor, and the intrinsic paradox of biomedicine (pharmaceutically synthesized drugs are expensive and not curing) we have to admit the failure of human kind: a failure in the battle against diabetes. This leads us to question: should we look another way? Look to Chinese medicine?

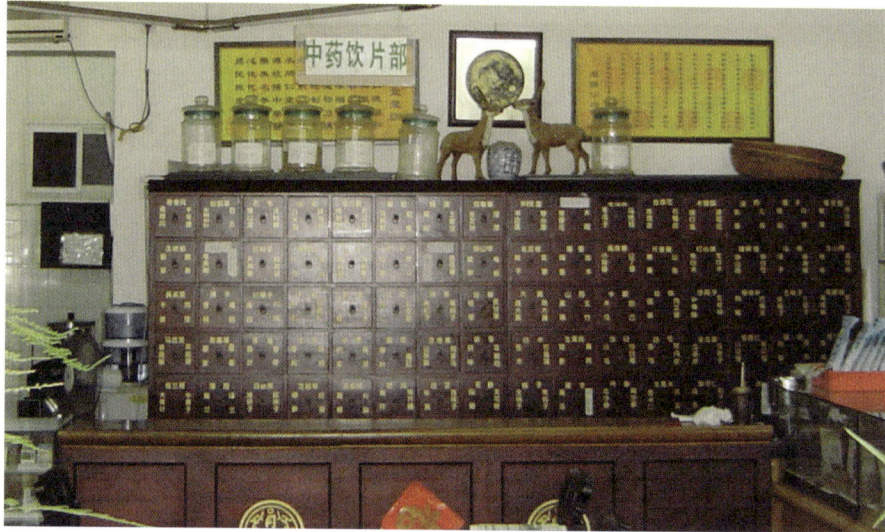

3. Additional Reading Material
(Disease Specific, General Chinese Medicine)

Chinese Medicine
- Xu Yi-bing. *An Illustrated Guide to* Chinese Medicine. People's Medical Publishing House, 2007
- Paul Pritchford. *Healing With Whole Foods: Asian Traditions and Modern Nutrition*. North Atlantic Books, 2003
- Harriet Beinfield, Efrem Korngold. *Between Heaven and Earth*. Random House, 1991
- Tom Williams. *Complete Illustrated Guide to* Chinese Medicine. Barnes & Noble INC, 1996
- Ted J. Kaptchuk. The Web That Has No Weaver Contemporary books, 2000
- http://www.acupuncture.com/education/tcmbasics/index.htm
- http://www.acupuncturetoday.com/abc/
- http://www.healthy.net/
- http://nccam.nih.gov/health/
- http://www.tcmstudent.com/
- http://www.nlm.nih.gov/hmd/chinese/chinesehome.html
- http://qi-journal.com/

Diabetes
- Janette Kirkham. *Mastering Your Diabetes; A Simple Plan for Taking Control of your Health.* American Diabetes Association, 2003
- Physicians Committee for Responsible Medicine. *Healthy Eating for Life to Prevent and Treat Diabetes.* Wiley, 2002
- William Polonsky. *Diabetes Burnout: What To Do When You Can't Take it Anymore.* American Diabetes Association. 1999
- Richard Bernstein. *Dr. Bernstein's Diabetes Solution: The Complete Guide to Achieving Normal Blood Sugars.* Little, Brown and Company, 2007
- http://www.answers.com/topic/diabetes-mellitus

Treatment of Diabetes with Chinese Medicine
- http://www.chinaqigong.net/english/tan.htm
- http://www.itmonline.org/journal/arts/diabetes.htm
- http://www.ontcm.com/dise/diab/main.htm
- http://www.chineseherbacademy.org/articles/dm2.shtml
- http://www.bluepoppy.com/press/featured/diabetes_chap.cfm
- http://diabetes.niddk.nih.gov/dm/pubs/diagnosis/
- http://www.newstarget.com/020606.html
- http://www.longevity-center.com/case_studies/48.html
- http://www.healthy.net/scr/article.asp?Id=3034
- http://www.chinesemedicinedoc.com/index.php?page=Chinese_Medicine_case_studies
- http://www.chinesemedicinedoc.com/index.php?page=108

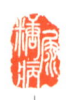

4. How to Find a Practitioner of Chinese Medicine?

Finding a practitioner of Chinese medicine is often as easy as looking in your local phone book. Most cities now have an "Acupuncture" heading in the yellow pages. Since acupuncture is the most well known modality of Chinese medicine in Western countries, those that practice Chinese herbalism will also be listed in this section. In many places, there will probably not be a practitioner who specializes in treating diabetes, but you may be able to find someone in the larger cities if you call around.

Most countries have established educational and license standards. A practitioner should be able to verify that these standards have been met.

The web can offer many ways to find a practitioner. Just searching for "acupuncture" and your town/area's name will probably locate something. The following internet resources should help you find a practitioner in your local area:

International Acupuncture Referral:
http://www.acufinder.com
http://www.gancao.net

Australia
Australian Acupuncture and Chinese Medicine Association
http://www.acupuncture.org.au

Canada
Traditional Chinese Medicine Association of British Columbia
http://tcmabc.org

Ordre des Acupuncteurs, Quebec
http://www.ordredesacupuncteurs.qc.ca

New Zealand
New Zealand Registrar of Acupuncture
http://acupuncture.org.nz

United Kingdom
Register of Chinese Herbal Medicine
http://www.rchm.cwww.acupuncture.org.uk
The British Medical Acupuncture Society
http://www.medical-acupuncture.co.uk

United States of America
National Certification Commission for Acupuncture and Oriental Medicine
http://nccaom.org
Council of Colleges of Acupuncture and Oriental Medicine
http://www.ccaom.org

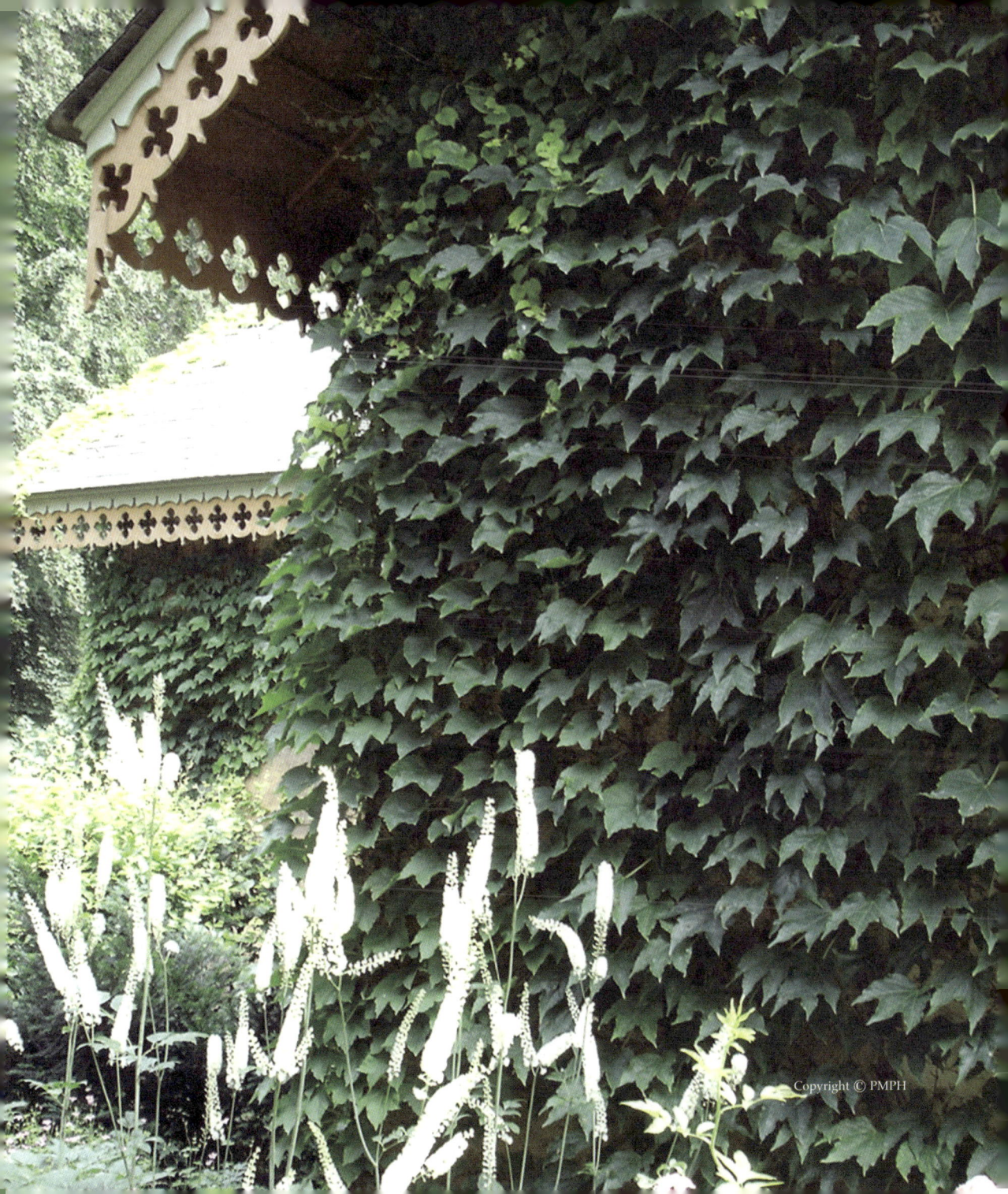

Reference

1. Kristen Philipkoski. Pigs May Hold Key To Diabetes. *Wired*. 2004, 2

2. Liu Tong-hua, Zheng Hong-yan. Essential Chinese Medical Dietary Therapy for Diabetes (糖尿病中医食疗述要). *International Journal Traditional Chinese Medicine (国际中医中药杂志)*. November 2006-Vo1 28. No 6

3. Xi Liu. Chinese Medicine Health and Dietary Therapy Forum (中国中医药论坛 养生食疗论坛). Retrieved on 2005/12/14 07:52pm from

4. http://www.cntm.org/cgi-bin/topic.cgi?forum=34&topic=226&show=175

5. Zinker. Nutrition and Exercise in Individuals with Diabetes. *Clinics in Sports Medicine*. 1999 18(3), 585-606.

6. Xin L, Miller YD, Brown WJ. A Qualitative Review of the Role of Qi Gong in the Management of Diabetes. *Journal of Alternative and Complementary Medicine*. 2007 May; 13(4): 427-33.

7. Iwao M, Kajiyama S, Mori H, Oogaki K. Effects of Qi gong Walking on Diabetic Patients: a Pilot Study. *Journal of Alternative and Complementary Medicine*. 1999 Aug;5(4):353-8.

8. Yeh SH, Chuang H, Lin LW, Hsiao CY, Wang PW, Yang KD. Tai Ji Quan Exercise Decreases A1C Levels Along With Increase of Regulatory T-cells and Decrease of Cytotoxic T-cell Population in Type 2 Diabetic Patients. *Diabetes Care*. 2007 Mar; 30(3):716-8.

9. Taylor-Piliae R, Haskell W, Stotts N, Froelicher E. Improvement in Balance, Strength, and Flexibility After 12 weeks of Tai Ji Exercise in Ethnic Chinese Adults With Cardiovascular Disease Risk Factors. *Alternative Therapy Health Medicine*. 2006 Mar-Apr; 12(2): 50-8.

10. Landt K, Campaigne B, James F, et al. Effects of Exercise Training on Insulin Sensitivity in Adolescents with Type I Diabetes. *Diabetes Care*. 1985 Sep-Oct; 8(5):461-5.

11. Wannamethee G, Sharper A. Physical Activity and Stroke in British Middle Aged Men. *British Medical Journal*. 1992 304(6827), 597-601

12. Uusitupa M, Louheranta A, Lindstrom J, Valle T, Sundvall J, Eriksson J, Tuomilehto J. The Finnish Diabetes Prevention Study. *British Journal of Nutrition*. 2000 83(Suppl. 1), S137-S142

13. Huang Xiaokuan. Medical Qi gong in the Treatment of Diabetes (医学气功治疗糖尿病的临床应用). *China Qi gong* (中国气功). 2000 (7)

14. Fu Shi-ming, Zhang Qing-mao, Zhang Xuan-xiang. Microcirculation Changes in the Qi gong Treatment of Diabetic Mice (糖尿病鼠在气功治疗过程中的微循环改变). *Oriental Qi gong* (东方气功) 1994 (1) 42

15. Qian Ai-zhu, Zhang Zhi-ying. Qi gong Treatment of 50 type II Diabetes (气功治疗2型糖尿病50例临床观察). *Shanghai Journal of Traditional Chinese Medicine* (上海中医药杂志). 1997 (10) 21-23

16. Yuan Shun-xing, Liu Wen-yong, Ding Xue-pin, et al. *Bu shen Qiang shen* Qi gong and Insulin Resistance in Type II Diabetes (补肾强身功对2型糖尿病胰岛素抵抗的影响). *Shanghai Journal of Traditional Chinese Medicine* (上海中医药杂志) 1999 v.1, p. 37-38

17. World Health Organization, Global Strategy on Diet, Physical Activity, and Health. *Diabetes*. www.who.int, 2003

18. Dong Jian-hua. *Case Records of Contemporary Prestigious Doctors of Chinese Medicine*. Beijing Publishing House, 1990 p. 1311 V2

19. Peter Sherwood. *Healing*. Australian College of Natural Medicine, 2006

20. Zhen Cheng. The Pandemic of Influenza Eighty Years Ago (80年前流感大流行). *Chinese Journal of Medical History* (中华医史杂志). No.4 1998

21. Molly Billings. The Influenza Pandemic of 1918. *http://virus.stanford.edu/uda/*, 1997

22. Huang Cong-qiang. Xie Jue-zai Enjoy's Support From Xiao ke Formula (谢觉哉喜赞"消渴"方). *Guangzhou Evening Edition* (羊城晚报). August 15, 2005

23. Ted J Kapchuk. *The Web that Has No Weaver*. Contemporary books, 2000

24. Xiao Qing-long. Shi Jin-mo Clinical Records: Diabetes (施今墨治消渴医案赏析) China Civil Network. Retrieved on 2006-12-28

13:31 from http://ngotcm.com/bbs/?action_viewthread_tid_39707.html

25. Yi Ming. Chinese Medicine in the Treatment of Diabetes (中医对糖尿病的治疗方法). Qianlong Net Chinese Medicine Report.

26. http://www.zgtnw.com/tnb/tnzl/zy/200703/3325.html

27. Zeng Zhi-yong, Li Yong-yi. Effect of pishu and zusanli on blood sugar and glucogon levels in diabetic rabbits (针刺胃脘下俞和足三里穴对糖尿病家兔血糖及血浆胰高血糖素的影响). *Journal of the Chengdu University of Chinese Medicine* (成都中医药大学学报). 2000 23(2) 40-41, 45

28. Zhang Yue-ping, Wang Xiang-yao, Li Cui-zhen. Histories of 73 Cases of Type 2 Diabetes Treated with Acupuncture (针刺治疗II型糖尿病73例临床观察). *Chinese Acupuncture and Moxibustion* (中国针灸). 1997, (11)673

29. Cao Shao-ming. A Comparative Study of Acupuncture, Moxibustion, and Acupuncture Plus Moxibustion in the Treatment of Diabetes (针刺、艾灸、针加灸治疗糖尿病的比较研究). *China Acupuncture and Moxibustion* (中国针灸). 1997 (10) 586-589

30. Liu Bao-hua, Li Yan-long. Use of Acupuncture Together with Chinese Herbal Medicine in the Treatment of Type II Diabetes: 30 Case Studies (针刺配合中药治疗2型糖尿病30例). *Journal of Clinical Acupuncture and Moxibustion* (针灸临床杂志). 2006 22 (7) 31-32

31. Liu Zhi-cheng, Sun Feng-min, Zhu Miaohua, et al. The Effect of Acupuncture on Insulin Resistance in Non Insulin-Dependent Diabetes Mellitus (针灸对非胰岛素依赖性糖尿病胰岛素抵抗的影响). *Shanghai Journal of Acupuncture and Moxibustion* (上海针灸杂志). 2000 19(1) 5-7

32. Qin Fu-lan, Jia Jie, Guo Xue-jun. Observation of the Therapeutic Effects of Acupuncture and Exercise Therapy on Type II Diabetes (针刺和运动疗法对2型糖尿病的疗效观察). *Chinese Acupuncture & Moxibustion* (中国针灸). 2002 22 (9) 579-581

33. Xiong Guang-yi, Wang Chun, Ouyang Hong. Effect of Acupuncture on Insulin Sensitivity Index of Type II Diabetes Mellitus (针刺对2型糖尿病胰岛素敏感指数的影响). *Journal of Yunnan College of Traditional Chinese Medicine* (云南中医学院学报). 2001 24(3) 38-39

34. Dong You-li, Zhu Sheng, Du Xueguang. Observation on the Therapeutic Effect

of Moxibustion Over Ginger as an Assistant Therapy to Treat Diabetes Mellitus Patients with Gastroparesis (隔姜施灸辅助治疗糖尿病胃轻瘫的效果观察). *Chinese Nursing Research* (护理研究). 2006 20 (7) 1897-1898

35. Han Gen-yan, Sun Hui. Effect of Warming Acupuncture on Diabetes Mellitus and Serum Corticosteroids (温针灸治疗糖尿病及其对血清皮质醇影响的观察). *Jiangsu Journal of Traditional Chinese Medicine* (江苏中医). 1996 17(1) 28

36. Zhang Ping, Liu Zhan-fen, Wang Chun-mei, et al. Observation on the Therapeutic Effect of Needling Method for Harmonizing Spleen-Stomach on Diabetic Gastroparesis (调理脾胃针法治疗糖尿病胃轻瘫疗效观察). *Chinese Acupuncture & Moxibustion* (中国针灸). 2007. 27 (4) 258-261

37. Zhang Shao-yun, Song Yi-hui, Li Bo-yi. Acupuncture and Medicinals in the Treatment of 60 Cases of Type II Diabetic Peripheral Neuropathy (针药结合治疗2型糖尿病末梢神经病变60例临床观察). *Yunnan Journal of Chinese Medicine* (云南中医中药杂志). 2006 27 (2) 33-34

38. Li Xu-jiong, Zhen Tian-zhen. Review of Chinese Medicinal in Lowering Blood Sugar Level (中药及其有效成分降血糖机制的研究进展). *Journal of Lanzhou University Medical Sciences* (兰州大学学报医). 2006 32(4)

39. Wang De-hui, Du Rui-bin, Zhou Qi. Effect of Chinese Herbal Medicine on Impaired Glucose Intolerance: An Observation (中药干预葡萄耐量低减的疗效观察). *Journal of Sichuan Traditional Chinese Medicine* (四川中医). 2006 24 (10) 63-64

40. Li Chang-chun. Chinese and Western Medicine Treat 80 Cases of Type II Diabetes (中西医结合治疗2型糖尿病80例). *New Journal of Traditional Chinese Medicine* (新中医). 2004 36 (11) 31

41. Deng De-qiang. Use of Supplementing the Spleen and Activating the Blood as a Treatment for Type II Diabetes Mellitus and Insulin Tolerance: a Clinical Study (培土活血解毒法治疗2型糖尿病及胰岛素抵抗的临床研究). *New Journal of Traditional Chinese Medicine* (新中医). 2003 35(4) 35-37

42. Shang Wen-bin, Jin Sha-wen. An Observation of Using of "Tang Keqing" as a Treatment of Non-insulin Dependent Diabetes Mellitus (糖渴清治疗非胰岛素依赖型糖尿病46例观察). *Traditional Chinese Medicinal Research* (中医研究). 1996 9(2) 26

43. Shang Wen-bin. Cheng Hai-bo, Si Xiao-chen, et al. Effect of Qing Zhi Jian Yi Capsule on Type II Diabetes Mellitus Insulin Tolerance Improvement (清脂健胰胶囊改善2型糖尿病胰岛素抵抗的研究). *Journal of Nanjing University of Traditional Chinese Medicine Natural Science* (南京中医药大学学报). 2003 19(4) 210-212

44. Chen Gang, Ni Yi--dong, Lai Xiao-ming, et al. Clinical Study on Xiaoke Pill in Treating Type II Diabetes Mellitus with Qi and Yin Deficiency (消渴丸治疗气阴两虚证2型糖尿病的临床研究). *Traditional Chinese Drug Research & Clinical Pharmacology* (中药新药与临床药理). 2003 14(2) 84

45. Yuan Xiao-han, Shi He-feng, Han Wei-feng. Use of Modified Artemisiae Capillariae Decoction as a Treatment of 40 Cases of Type II Diabetes Mellitus (加味茵陈蒿汤治疗2型糖尿病40例). *Traditional Chinese Medicinal Research* (中医研究). 20(2) 43

46. Lin Mei. Chinese and Western Medicine Used Together on Diabetes Mellitus: A Clinical Observation (中西医结合治疗糖尿病38例观察). *Journal of Sichuan Traditional Chinese Medicine* (四川中医). 2004 22(2) 38

47. Du Yu-ke, Wang Juan-wen. Use of San Se Powder and Western Medicine as Treatment of 56 Cases of Diabetes Mellitus (中药三色散配合西药降糖药治疗糖尿病56例). *Shaanxi Journal of Traditional Chinese Medicine* (陕西中医). 2004 25(10) 885-886

48. Chen Ze-qi, Liu Xiao-zhen, Chen Da-shun. Observation of the Clinical Efficacy of Prescriptions of Traditional Chinese Medicine in 60 Cases of Type II Diabetes (中医传统方为主治疗2型糖尿病60例临床疗效观察). *Journal of Chinese Physicians* (中国医师杂志). 2006 8(8) 1035-1037

49. Lin Chen. Use of Chinese and Western Medicine as Treatment of Qi and Yin Deficiency Diabetes Mellitus 35 Cases (中西医结合治疗气阴两虚型老年性糖尿病35例). *Fujian Journal of Traditional Chinese Medicine* (福建中医药). 2000 31(4) 12-14

50. Mehrotra R, Bajaj S., Kumar D. Use of Complementary and Alternative Medicine by Patients with Diabetes Mellitus. *Natural Medicine Journal of India*. 2004 Sep-Oct;17(5):243-5.

51. Zhang Zhi-yong, Li Zhen-hua. Tui na Treatment of 30 Cases of Type II Diabetes (推拿治疗2型糖尿病30例). *Jilin Chinese Medicinal Journal* (吉林中医药). 2006.11.26.11

52. Zhang Jia-fu. Analysis of Tui na Treat-

ment of Type II Diabetes (推拿治疗2型糖尿病疗效分析). *Chinese Journal of Clinical Rehabilitation (中国临床康复)*. 2003.1.15 no.7, volume 1

53. Cui Ren-ming, Zhu Bian. *An Illustrated Guide to Diabetes (图说糖尿病)*. People's Medical Publishing House. 2006

54. Pan Yun-hua, Geng Tao. Tui na and Type II Diabetes: a Case Report (耿涛.推拿治疗2型糖尿病患者1例). *Modern Journal of Integrated Traditional Chinese and Western Medicine (现代中西医结合杂志)*. 2003,12(23):2 562—2563.

55. Zhang Jia-fu. Tui na and Type II Diabetes: a Controlled Clinical Trial (章家福推拿治疗2型糖尿病疗效分析). *Chinese Journal of Clinical Rehabilitation (中国临床康复)*. 2003 7 (1)

56. Yu Zhao-hua, Yu Wei-jie, Li Tie-shan, Chen Fu-xiang, Liu Chang-chang. Short-term Curative Effect of Traditional Massage on Type II Diabetes Mellitus (推拿按脊治疗2型糖尿病近期疗效分析). *China Journal of Clinical Rehabilitation (中国临床康复)*. 2006.R10(39):30- 2

57. Zhou Zhao. Treatment of 72 Cases of Diabetes with Tui Na (推拿治疗糖尿病72例临床分析). *Hunan Journal of Chinese Medicine (湖南中医药导报)*. 2003. June 9-6

58. Wen Ling. Tui Na Treatment of 76 Cases of Diabetic Peripheral Neuropathy (推拿治疗糖尿病周围神经病变76例). *Chinese Cardiovascular and Cerebrovascular Journal of Integrative Medicine*. 2006 (4) 366

59. Yu Qi, Shao Xue-ying, Hu Li-zhen. The Effect of Foot Massage on the Treatment of Diabetic Peripheral Neuropathy (足穴推拿治疗糖尿病周围神经病变的疗效观察). *China Journal of Science and Technology (中国中医药科技)*. 2005. Sept. (12)5 p.325 ·

60. Personal account by Jiang Miao, postgraduate student of Chinese Medicine

61. Zhao Jin-xi. *Treatment of Endocrine and Metabolic Diseases with Western and Chinese Medicine (内分泌代谢病中西医诊治)*. Liaoning Science and Technology Publishing House. 2004, p153

62. Zhang Yong-long, Wang Guang-yi. Treatment of Kidney Disease in 38 Diabetes Patients with Chinese Medicine and Biomedicine (中西医结合治疗糖尿病肾病28例). *Guiyang Medical University Journal (贵阳医学院学报)*. 2001 no.5

63. Lin Chen. Use of Chinese Medicine and Biomedicine as Treatment of Qi and Yin Deficiency Diabetes Mellitus, 35 Cases (中西医结合治疗气阴两虚型糖尿病35例). *Fujian Journal of Traditional Chinese Medicine* (福建中医学院学报). 2000 31(4) 12

64. Renming, Zhu Bian. *An Illustrated Guide to Diabetes* (图说糖尿病). People's Medical Publishing House. 2006

65. Deadman, Peter, Al-Khafaji, Mazin. *A Manual of Acupuncture.* Journal of Chinese Medicine Press. 2006

66. Kapchuk, Ted. *The Web that Has No Weaver.* Contemporary books. 2000

67. Stonefoot, Sarah, Freeman, Clyde. A Need for Needles, Acupuncture - Does it Really Work? Herreid University at Buffalo. 2004 http://www.sciencecases.org/acupuncture/acupuncture_notes.asp

68. Wiseman, Nigel, Ellis, Andrew. *Fundamentals of Chinese Medicine*, Paradigm Publications. 1996

69. Wu Den Xu. *Basic Theories of Chinese Medicine* (中医基础理论). Shanghai Science and Technology Publishing House. 1996

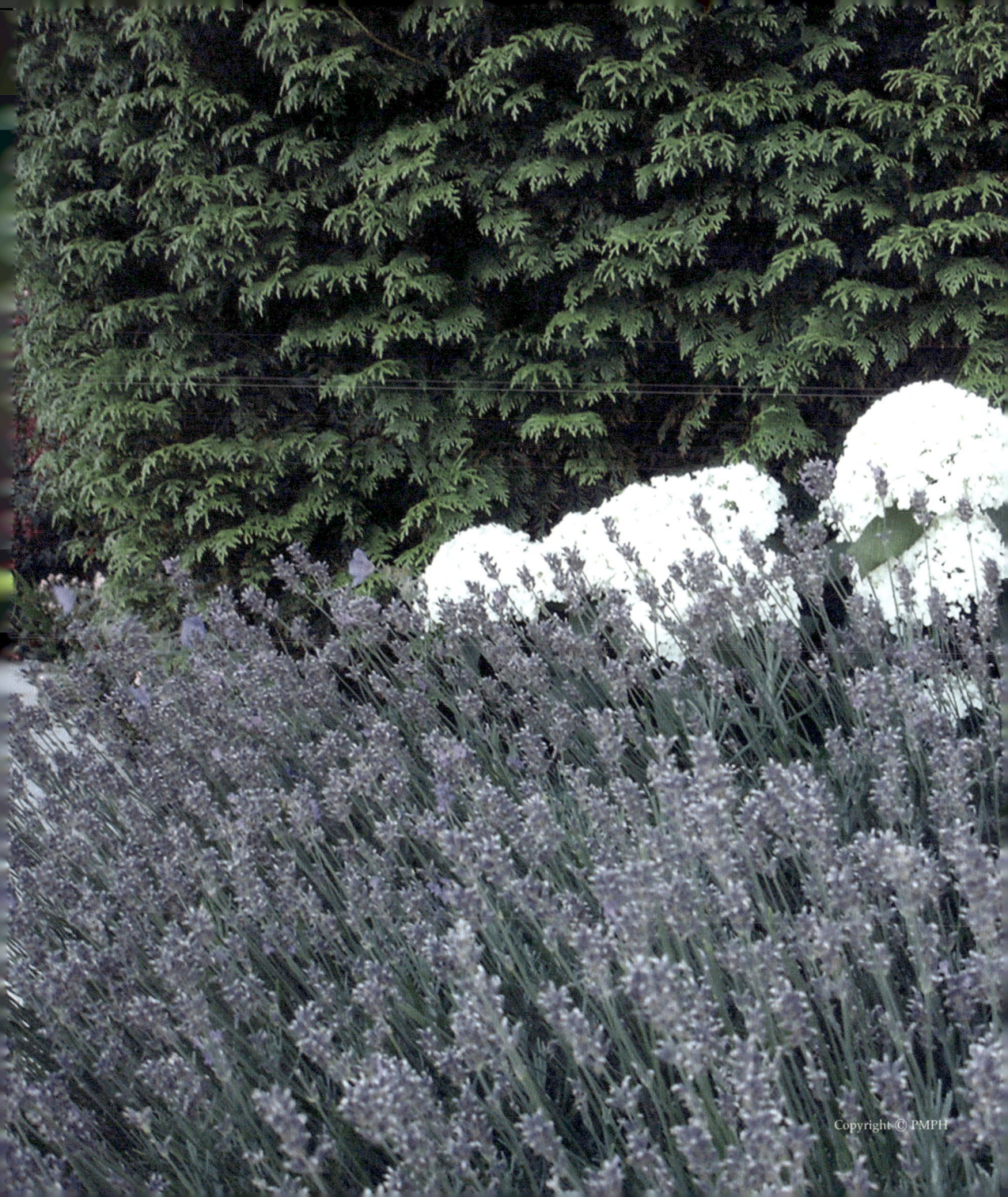

Index

A

Acupuncture 4,21,64,70,71,73,76,87,100
acupuncture needle 74,81
acupuncture & moxibustion 71
acupressure 112
alcohol 44
amorphophallus Konjac 46
antibodies 73
astragalus 20,21
astragalus-polysaccharides 21
asthma 81
anti-symptomatic 92
anti-diabetic 107

B

Biàn Zhèng Lùn Zhì 32
bitter melon 44,45
blood 13,31,72,90
blood cell 73
biomedicine 8,12,20
blood sugar 7
buffer 81
blister 81

C

carbohydrates 41
channels & collaterals (jing luo) 72
Chinese White and Black Fungus 46
chyluria 30
Clean Needle Technique 74
coix seed 46
complication 30
Chinese medicinal 64,90

cupping 82,84,86,100
chronic disease 102
chéng jiāng 118
central stomach cavity 118
channel theory 124

D

dān tián 63,117,120
decoction 101,102,108
dé qì 85,86
dì huáng 93
dì gǔ pí 97
diabetic ketoacidosis 83
direct moxabustion 80
diabetic neuropathy 108
diabetic retinopathy 32
diabetic skin infection 83
diet 41
duck 44

E

ear acupuncture 82
eel 47
electroacupuncture 75
Elixir Field 117
energy tonic 94
essence 96

F

fat 42
fatigue 20,83
Five element theory 27

G

garlic 44,81
gauze 108
gě gēn 98
ginger 44,81
ginseng *(rén shēn)* 20
gold needle 74
Gold Theragran 45
goose 44
gǒu qǐ zǐ 93,97
gou Qi Berries 93
granule 107
guān yuán 78,119

H

herb 92
herbal 100
herbal formula 100
Herbal King 105
herbal medication 70
hot spices 44
huáng dì nèi jīng 18
huáng lián 92,98
huáng qí 93,95
huáng jīng 96,97
hyperosmolar coma 83
hypodermic needles 85

I

immune response 73
indirect moxibustion 81
innate ability 7
insomnia 71
insulin 7,41
internal heat 107
invaluable Prescriptions for Emergencies (Bèi Jí Qiān Jīn Yào Fāng) 76

J

jingluo 12,124

K

kidney 78
kidney yang 28
kiwi 44

L

liver 78
Lower xiao 34

M

massage 21
medication 41
mental stress 83
metabolic disorder 83
Middle xiao 34
milk 44
millet 44
Miscellaneous Recors of Famous (míng Yī Bié Lù) 79
moxa 81,84,86
moxa cone 81
moxa pole 81
moxibustion 21,64,70,71,73,79,80,88,100
mushroom 46

N

needle 72,84
nèi guān 116
neurotransmitter 73
non-herbal medication 70
numbness 33
nurturing 19

O
obtaining the qi 85

P
pancreas 125
pattern *(Zhèng)* 32
pí shù 77
physicians 79
pig pancreas 47
plucking 85
plum-blossom needling 82
Pneuma 15
points *(xué wèi)* 72
pork 52
Protein 42

Q
qi 8,13,14,15,16,17,18,19,27,31,32,72,76,77,90,111
qi deficiency 32
qi gong 57,61,62,64
qī mén 119
qi of the kidney 21
qi of the lung 21
qi of spleen (pancreas) 21
Qi-transforming 19

R
rabbit 44
raising 85
Records of Proven Formulas Past and Present (Gǔ Jīn Lù Yàn) 30
Reflexology 124
Rén shēn 94
re-trained 8
Royal Jelly 47

S
salt 81
sān yīn jiāo 78
sāng bái pí 99
saponin 21
scars 81
scraping 85
sea cucumber 44
self-massage 114
Senna Leaf 52
shén mén 78
Shen Nong's Herbal *(Shén Nóng Běn Cǎo Jīng)* 79
shèn shù 120
shen xiao 30
Shēng Mài Sǎn 104,107
shēng (shú) dì huáng 95
shortness of breath 20
shou fa 113
shù 77
side-effect 6,73
silver needle 74
spicy food 44
spinach 44
spirits 12
spirit gate 78
spleen 78
spleen transport 77
sweating 20
symptom 7
syndrome of thirst 30
synthesized drug 73

T
tai ji 4,57,58,60,61,62
tea 52

techniques of the hands 113
the Sea of Yin 78
thrusting 85
tiān huā fěn 99
tomato 44
triglyceride 73
tui na 70,111,112,113,114
turnip 44
twirling 85
type I 6
type II 6

U

ulcer 83
upper *xiao* 34

V

vitamins 42

W

water chestnut 44
Water Spinach 45
weakness of qi 20
white gourd 44

X

xiao ke 30,33,76

xiao ke bing 134
xiao zhong 30
Xī Yáng Shēn 94
xuán shēn 96

Y

yam 44
yang 13,14,23,24,25,26,28,31,76,90
yang deficiency 26,32
Yellow Emperor's Classic of Internal Medicine (Huáng Dì Nèi Jīng) 18,29,38
yí 77
yí shù 76,77
yin 13,14,23,24,25,26,28,31,32,76 ,90
yin deficiency 32, 48
yin excess 26
yin organs 78
yin-yang 8,27,79
yin-yang imbalance 26
yin-yang theory 4,22

Z

zhen Jiu 71
zú sān lǐ 76,77
zhōng wǎn 118

图书在版编目（CIP）数据

中医科普系列——糖尿病（英文）/李晓莉等主编．—北京：
人民卫生出版社，2008.3
 ISBN 978-7-117-09119-0

Ⅰ.中… Ⅱ.李… Ⅲ.糖尿病－中医治疗法－英文
Ⅳ.R259.871

中国版本图书馆 CIP 数据核字（2007）第 123331 号

中医科普系列——糖尿病
（英文）

主　　编：	李晓莉　卡尔·斯蒂姆森
出版发行：	人民卫生出版社（中继线＋8610-6761-6688）
地　　址：	北京市丰台区方庄芳群园三区 3 号楼
邮　　编：	100078
网　　址：	http://www.pmph.com
E－mail：	pmph @ pmph.com
发　　行：	zzg@pmph.com.cn
够书热线：	＋8610-6769-1034（电话及传真）
开　　本：	850×1168　1/24
版　　次：	2008 年 3 月第 1 版　2008 年 3 月第 1 版第 1 次印刷
标准书号：	ISBN 978-7-117-09119-0/R·9120

版权所有，侵权必究，打击盗版举报电话：＋8610-8761-3394
（凡属印装质量问题请与本社销售部联系退换）